Radiotherap
Cancer Management

JOIN US ON THE INTERNET VIA WWW, GOPHER, FTP OR EMAIL:

WWW: http://www.thomson.com
GOPHER: gopher.thomson.com
FTP: ftp.thomson.com
EMAIL: findit@kiosk.thomson.com

A service of I(T)P

Radiotherapy in Cancer Management

A practical manual

**Published on behalf of
the World Health Organization**

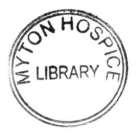

CHAPMAN & HALL MEDICAL

London · Weinheim · New York · Tokyo · Melbourne · Madras

Published by Chapman & Hall, 2–6 Boundary Row, London SE1 8HN, UK

Chapman & Hall, 2–6 Boundary Row, London SE1 8HN, UK

Chapman & Hall GmbH, Pappelallee 3, 69469 Weinheim, Germany

Chapman & Hall USA, 115 Fifth Avenue, New York, NY 10003, USA

Chapman & Hall Japan, ITP-Japan, Kyowa Building, 3F, 2–2–1 Hirakawacho, Chiyoda-ku, Tokyo 102, Japan

Chapman & Hall Australia, 102 Dodds Street, South Melbourne, Victoria 3205, Australia

Chapman & Hall India, R. Seshadri, 32 Second Main Road, CIT East, Madras 600 035, India

First edition 1997

© 1997 The World Health Organization

Typeset in 10/12 Times by Photoprint, Torquay
Printed in Great Britain at the University Press, Cambridge

ISBN 0 412 63580 1

A catalogue record for this book is available from the British Library

♾ Printed on permanent acid-free text paper, manufactured in accordance with ANSI/NISO Z39.48–1992 and ANSI/NISO Z39.48–1981 (Permanence of Paper).

Contents

Contributors

This manual has been prepared by the members of the WHO Working Group on Radiation Therapy in Cancer. WHO wishes particularly to acknowledge the contributions of Professor C.F. von Essen and Dr. M.K. Nair to the editing of the text and of Professor J.P. Gérard and Dr I. Marquis to the preparation of the illustrations and treatment plans.

Francis Durosinmi-Etti, International Atomic Energy Agency, Vienna, Austria

Schmuel El-Haddad, Kaar El-Einy Center for Oncology and Nuclear Medicine, Manial University Hospital, Cairo, Egypt

Carl F. von Essen, Departments of Radiation Medicine, Southwood Community Hospital, Norfolk, and Massachusetts General Hospital, Boston, Massachusetts, USA

Jean-Pierre Gérard, Service de Radiothérapie, Centre Hospitalier Lyon-Sud, France

Gerald P. Hanson, Radiation Medicine, World Health Organization, Geneva, Switzerland

Alan Horwich, Section of Radiotherapy, The Institute of Cancer Research and the Royal Marsden Hospital, Sutton, Surrey, UK

Nora Janjan, Department of Radiation Therapy, M.D. Anderson Hospital, Houston, Texas, USA

Jeff Luande, Tanzania Tumour Centre, Dar-es-Salaam, United Republic of Tanzania

Isabelle Marquis, Service de Radiothérapie, Polyclinique de Gentilly, Nancy, France

W.M. Craig Martin, Radiotherapy Department, Parirenyatwa Hospital, Harare, Zimbabwe (currently at Department of Clinical Oncology, Norfolk and Norwich Hospital, UK)

M. Krishna Nair, Regional Cancer Centre, Trivandrum, India

David Otim-Oyet, Radiotherapy Department, Parirenyatwa Hospital, Harare, Zimbabwe

Luis Souhami, Department of Radiation Oncology, McGill University, Montreal, Canada

Jan Stjernswärd, Cancer and Palliative Care, World Health Organization, Geneva, Switzerland

Yang Tian-En, Department of Radiation Oncology, Tianjin Medical College, Tianjin, China

Preface

Standard therapies can cure many patients provided cancers are diagnosed early and basic therapies are available. However, for years to come, the majority of the world's cancer patients will be incurable, mainly due to late diagnosis. Attention must therefore be given not only to curative treatment but also to palliative care. Radiotherapy is a modality that offers benefits to patients in many situations, both as curative and as palliative therapy.

Radiotherapy is the backbone of most cancer care, and in many countries the radiotherapist is the only cancer specialist. To be really effective, the radiotherapist cannot afford to be only a 'super-technician'. It is also the radiotherapist's responsibility to help develop programmes that will lead to earlier diagnosis as well as to provide pain relief and palliative care.

Earlier referral of many common cancers such as those of the cervix uteri, breast and mouth has greater prognostic importance than any therapeutic efforts, however sophisticated, as shown in the following table.

	In developed countries		In developing countries	
Stage of disease at diagnosis	Percentage of patients	Five-year survival	Percentage of patients	Action required
I–II	~80% →	80%	< 20%	Earlier referral and diagnosis to ensure that 80% of patients are stage I or II (as in developed countries)
III–IV	~20%	20%	> 80%	

Ideally, the radiotherapist, trained to deal with cancer in almost any site, has the potential for leadership in regional and national cancer control programmes, and should address not only therapy, but also prevention, earlier referral and palliative care. In the near future, two-thirds of cancer patients will be in developing countries, but with only 5% of the global resources for cancer control. Thus therapy should not be addressed in isolation, and readers are urged to read the WHO publication *National Cancer Control Programmes. Priorities and Managerial Guidelines* (1995).

A practical handbook of radiotherapy is needed, however, for use in the frontlines of the battle against cancer. It should be easily available at the critical time when a cancer patient is first seen in the clinic. This manual provides concise and useful information about incidence and risk factors, the natural history, the necessary diagnostic investigations and the staging of the cancer which can aid the physician in vital management decisions. These decisions include whether to pursue a radical and curative treatment policy or to provide palliative care and supportive management.

From these decisions, specific methods of treatment can then be formulated. No manual or single-volume textbook can hope to describe in enough detail all the treatments that are possible in all circumstances. Therefore, this manual provides examples of the basic radiotherapeutic approaches to treatment. Other modalities, including chemotherapy and hormonal therapy, are mentioned when appropriate. Since the majority of cancer patients worldwide present to the medical clinic at a stage that is beyond hope of cure, palliative treatment methods are discussed.

This manual was written by expert radiation oncologists from all parts of the world. Their experience is brought together in an attempt to achieve a consensus regarding the issues mentioned above. No absolute consensus is possible with such markedly divergent experiences. However, it is hoped that the information provided is of practical use and will support the frontline radiotherapist in the daily task of coping with the diverse problems presented by cancer patients.

Various techniques, including the use of cobalt-60 teletherapy units as well as of linear accelerators, are presented and sometimes compared in order to provide information for those facilities relying on telecobalt.

The introductory chapter regarding the organization of radiotherapy facilities and regional needs for radiotherapy resources will also be useful for national health and hospital administrators. A review of clinical fundamentals leads to chapters on site-specific management. A list of useful references focusing on general issues is provided.

This manual is intended to be complementary and interdependent with existing textbooks on oncology and radiotherapy.

Jan Stjernswärd MD, PhD
Former Chief, Cancer and Palliative Care,
World Health Organization

Gerald P. Hanson Dr.PH
Former Chief, Radiation Medicine, World Health Organization

Treatment plans and isodose distributions: note on interpretation

Treatment plans and isodose distributions have been displayed in a uniform way throughout the manual. The treatment plan always illustrates a technique described in the corresponding chapter. The treatment techniques using cobalt-60 are based on source-to-skin technique with a source-to skin distance (SSD) of 80 cm, while the treatment techniques using X-rays produced by a linear accelerator are based on isocentric techniques involving the source–axis distance (SAD), which is 100 cm for most modern accelerators. Nevertheless, in clinical practice, it is possible to use a cobalt-60 unit for isocentric techniques and to use a linear accelerator for source-to-skin techniques.

The contours are based on a standard patient. The isodoses have been plotted with a TPS 2 Philips computer and program. The isodoses are normalized (100%) usually on the ICRU point in the centre of the planned target volume. The maximum dose in the irradiated area is usually mentioned as is the 95% isodose which encompasses the treated volume. Wedges are identified by a triangle. The isodoses displayed are usually 25, 50, 80, 95, 100 and 105%.

DEFINITIONS

SAD	Source–axis distance
SSD	Source–skin distance
AP	Anterior–posterior
PA	Posterior–anterior

1

Modalities, resources and organization

1.1 MODALITIES FOR RADIOTHERAPY

Ideally, modalities should be available for treating all types of tumours, ranging from superficial lesions of the skin to deep-seated tumours and for curative as well as palliative objectives. The various radiotherapeutic modalities may be classified in several ways: by the location of the radiation source (either external or internal to the patient's body), by the ability of the radiation to penetrate tissue (e.g. as a function of the generating potential or the energy of the radiation), by the type of radiation (e.g. photons, electrons, neutrons, protons, heavy nuclei), and by the method of production of the radiation (e.g. by an electrical machine or by the disintegration of a radionuclide).

1.1.1 External beam therapy

For external beam therapy the various radiation sources, classified according to the energy of the radiation, and their use for cancer treatment are shown in Table 1.1.

Medium-energy (orthovoltage) radiograph machines with generating potentials in the range 100–300 kV which originally were used to treat deep-seated tumours are no longer recommended for that purpose, having been replaced by 'megavoltage' machines operating at effective energies equal to or above the energy of telecobalt (1.25 MV). The advantages of higher energy radiation that are now universally accepted are:

Table 1.1 External beam therapy sources, classified by their energy and their use for cancer treatment

Type of equipment	Generating potential of energy	Type of radiation	Use and comment
Contact therapy machines	10–60 kV	X-ray	Treatment of skin lesions. Seldom used
Low-voltage (superficial) X-ray machines	below 100 kV	X-ray	Treatment of superficial lesions immediately beneath the skin. Useful and recommended for every radiotherapy centre
Medium-voltage (orthovoltage) X-ray machines	100–300 kV	X-ray	Treatment of lesions a few centimetres beneath the surface. Seldom used and not recommended
Beta-ray applicators	540 keV (Sr 90)	Beta rays (electrons)	Treatment of superficial lesions and eye malignancies. Seldom used
Caesium-137	660 keV	Gamma ray	Treatment of lesions up to some centimetres beneath the surface. Not recommended
Cobalt-60	1.25 MeV (mean)	Gamma ray	Treatment of medium and deep-seated tumours. Very useful and highly recommended
Low-energy accelerators (< 8 MV)			
Photon beams only, no electron beams	4–6 MV (common use)	X-ray	Not recommended in developing countries. No significant difference from cobalt-60, and more complicated accelerators
Medium-energy accelerators (≥ 8 MV)			
Photon beams	8–20 MV (common use)	X-ray	Treatment of deep-seated tumours. Useful in appropriate circumstances

Table 1.1 Continued

Type of equipment	Generating potential of energy	Type of radiation	Use and comment
Electron beams	6–20 MeV (common use)	Electrons	Treatment of lesions a few centimetres (perhaps up to 6 cm) beneath the surface. Useful in appropriate circumstances
High-energy accelerators (> 20 MV)			
Photon beams	5–50 MV (available)	X-rays	Treatment of deep-seated tumours. Useful in appropriate circumstances
Electron beams	5–50 MeV (available)	Electrons	Treatment of lesions approximately 1–13 cm beneath the surface

- the skin-sparing effect due to the build-up of electrons below the surface;
- the greater power of penetration and hence the increased percentage depth–dose;
- the decreased scatter sideways from the direction of the beam and consequently sharper delineation of the beam;
- smaller increase in specific absorption in bone compared to soft tissue.

Figure 1.1 shows typical depth–dose curves on the central axis of the radiation beam for (a) photons and (b) electrons of various energies. Depth–dose curves show the percentage of the absorbed dose at a given depth within a substance (usually water or another tissue-like material) compared to its maximum value (100%) at another point within the substance. For high-energy radiation, the point of maximum dose may range from several millimetres to several centimetres below the surface. Beyond the point of maximum dose, the percentage of the absorbed dose for radiation gradually decreases with increasing depth. For electrons, the shape of the curves is quite different, with only a small build-up between the surface and the point of maximum value (100%), and then a

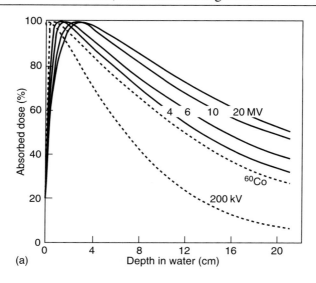

(a)

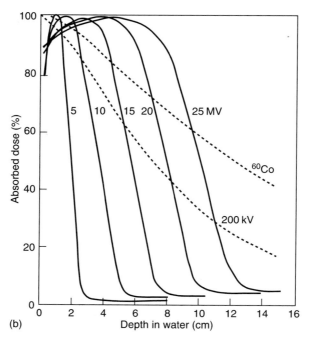

(b)

Figure 1.1 Depth–dose curves for (a) photons and (b) electrons.

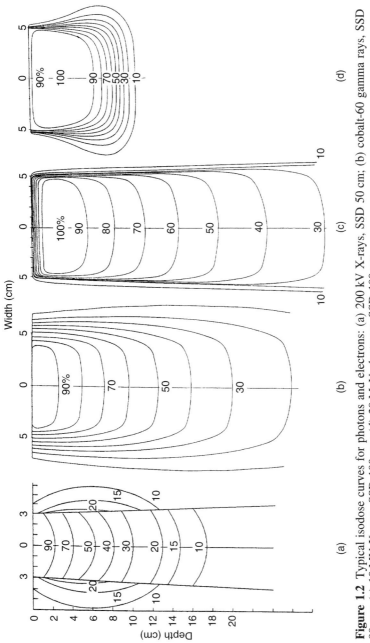

Figure 1.2 Typical isodose curves for photons and electrons: (a) 200 kV X-rays, SSD 50 cm; (b) cobalt-60 gamma rays, SSD 80 cm; (c) 10 MV X-rays, SSD 100 cm; (d) 20 MeV electrons, SSD 100 cm.

sharply decreasing percentage of dose to almost zero at a relatively short distance from the maximum.

Figure 1.2 shows typical isodose curves for the radiation beams of photons and electrons of various energies. Isodose curves join the depths within a substance being irradiated that have received the same absorbed dose.

The practical implications of the physical difference in the dose distributions of photons compared to electrons can be appreciated from the curves of Figures 1.1 and 1.2.

For the treatment of tumours which extend from the surface to a depth of several centimetres, electron beam therapy allows a high dose to be given to the tumour while the dose to healthy tissue at a greater depth is very low (nearly zero). Thus where curative therapy is attempted, high-energy electron beams are an important modality for irradiating the chest wall after mastectomy, treating posterior cervical nodes over the spinal cord, reducing the dose to the heart during treatment of internal mammary nodes, and 'boosting' doses to intra-oral and pharyngeal tumours.

However, for deep-seated tumours, at a depth of more than 8–10 cm below the surface, high-energy electrons have not been shown to have an advantage over high-energy photons. For treatment of these kinds of tumours, very high-energy electrons of at least 30 MeV would be needed with two opposing fields. Very few accelerators for radiotherapy with such energies are in use today. The treatment situation often used for deep-seated tumours consists of two opposing photon fields. The following table can be constructed giving the maximum acceptable thickness of tissue between the opposing fields.

Type of photon radiation	Maximum distance between fields (cm)
250 kV	16
Telecobalt	23
4 MV	27
8 MV	34

With regard to external beam therapy, the following points should be considered in deciding on the necessary compromise for providing the treatment machines.

(a) Accelerators

Advantages

1. Sharper beam delineation (smaller physical penumbra than telecobalt).
2. Higher radiation output than telecobalt.
3. Higher penetration of photons in tissue than telecobalt: photons of 4–6 MV have only moderately higher penetration than telecobalt while higher photon energies (over 6 MV) often give some advantages in deep-seated tumours.
4. Greater ease in treating large patients and lesions that are difficult to treat because of size, shape or location (may be 10–15% of all patients treated).
5. Units are available which can produce electron beams: if purchase is being considered, an electron beam of variable energy up to about 20 MeV covers most applications.

Requirements

1. Extensive resources for the initial purchase and for construction of the treatment room.
2. Reliable electricity supply, not subject to voltage reductions or interruptions.
3. Availability of good service from the manufacturer or supplier, including spare parts locally available, and easy access to telephone communication.
4. Excellent radiation dosimetry and quality assurance capabilities in the department.
5. Well-trained staff especially qualified to work with high-energy photons and electrons: a very sharp beam delineation can only be fully exploited if the rest of the treatment procedure is very accurate, e.g. accurate diagnostic outlining of the tumour volume and careful setting-up and positioning of the patient.

(b) Telecobalt teletherapy machine

Advantages

1. Provides high-energy photons (average 1.25 MeV).
2. Many years of experience in the use of these units has proven their dependability.

3. Adequate dose distributions can be obtained for most practical treatment situations.
4. The initial capital investment and routine operating costs are moderate.
5. Installation can be achieved in a relatively short time with moderately skilled workers.
6. Few total staff required, and staff with moderate levels of training are sufficient for routine operation.
7. Maintenance and repair are not required frequently and when needed are moderate in cost.

Requirements

1. Adequate premises and shielding must be provided.
2. Provision must be made for replacement of the telecobalt source at periodic intervals.
3. Trained staff in sufficient numbers are necessary.
4. For curative treatment of certain cancers (e.g. very deep-seated lesions or lesions near critical tissues), more care in planning is required (as compared to accelerators) because of the less penetrating radiation and the larger penumbra.

As an example of the need for additional attention to treatment planning needed when using telecobalt, the more complex beam arrangement utilizing more than two opposing fields is considered below. The table shows the maximum depth for three fields for various types of photon beams.

Type of photon radiation	Maximum depth (cm) for three fields	Maximum depth (cm) for four fields
250 kV	6.5	9.5
Telecobalt	11.5	15.5
4 MV	13.5	18
8 MV	17	22

1.1.2 Internal therapy

Treatment with radioisotopes used internally may be classified as therapy using sealed radioactive sources (brachytherapy) or un-

Table 1.2 Radioisotopes used as sealed sources for internal radiotherapy

Radioisotope source	Half life	Energy (McV)		Principal uses and comment
		Beta	Gamma	
Caesium-137	30 years	0.51	0.66	Removable interstitial implants and intracavitary insertion
Cobalt-60	5.27 years	0.31	1.17–1.33	Removable interstitial implants, intracavitary insertion, surface application
Gold-198	2.7 days	0.96	0.41	Permanent interstitial implants
Iridium-192	74.4 days	0.57	0.30–0.61	Removable interstitial implants
Radium-226	1622 years	3.17	0.18–2.20	Interstitial implants and intracavitary insertion. Not recommended because of its potential hazard
Radon-222	3.8 days	3.17	0.18–2.20	Permanent interstitial implants
Strontium-90	28 years	0.2		Surface applications
Tantalum-182	11.5 days		0.07–1.2	Interstitial implants
Yttrium-90	64 h	0.93		Interstitial implants

sealed radioactive sources (systemic therapy). Brachytherapy is used for intracavitary spaces (principally cancer of the cervix and corpus uteri, although it may also be useful in treatment of cancer of the oesophagus), for interstitial implants within tissues (e.g. for cancers of the breast and tongue), and for surface treatment of accessible tumours. Radiotherapy with unsealed sources has a rather limited role, principally being used for thyroid disorders, polycythaemia vera, and for cancers within the peritoneal cavity.

In developing countries, the most beneficial use of internal therapy is for treatment of cancer of the cervix. For internal radiotherapy the sealed radiation sources are shown in Table 1.2 and the unsealed sources in Table 1.3.

Table 1.3 Radioisotopes used as unsealed sources for internal radiotherapy

Radioisotope source	Half life	Energy (McV)		Principal uses and comment
		Beta	Gamma	
Gold-198	2.7 days	0.32 (mean)	0.41	Colloidal suspension for intracavitary or interstitial application. Less economical than phosphorus-32 or yttrium-90, and has no proven therapeutic advantage
Iodine-131	8 days	0.19 (mean)	0.08–0.72 (mean 0.284)	Oral solution for systemic use, e.g. thyroid cancer, hyperthyroidism
Phosphorus-32	14.3 days	0.69 (mean)	–	Oral and injectable solution, e.g. for polycythaemia vera
Yttrium-90	64 h	0.93 (mean)		Injectable solution
Strontium-89	50.5 days	0.58 (mean)		Injectable solution

1.2 RESOURCES FOR RADIOTHERAPY

The resources needed for radiotherapy can be classified as human resources (radiotherapy department staff, plus collaborating staff from other clinical departments), equipment or physical premises (the radiotherapy department plus the structures housing other supporting services, and facilities for the hospitalization or lodging of patients). The extent of the resources needed within the main categories will depend on the functions to be performed. The functions performed in any specific radiotherapy department (including its peripheral supporting clinical departments or services) will depend on the level of services provided and these may range from essential clinical treatment services for patients to teaching and research serving the broader interests of society. Conceptually, three levels of services can be identified as described below, although in practice there may be intermediate levels and overlapping.

1.2.1 Level 1: essential radiotherapy department

At level 1, the principal objective is the provision of essential radiotherapy services for the clinical management and treatment of patients. Most of the treatments will be for cancer, with some benign diseases being treated depending on the local pathology. There will be little or no effort devoted to teaching or research, although the staff may be involved in the collection and analysis of epidemiological data concerning local disease patterns and in the provision of information concerning prevention of cancer.

1.2.2 Level 2: comprehensive radiotherapy department

The same types of activities will be conducted as in a level 1 department, although the level of sophistication and ambition will be increased due to the existence of more complex equipment and a wider range of staff expertise. In addition, training for radiation oncologists, physicists, radiation therapy technologists and other supporting staff may be provided. Clinical research will be conducted.

1.2.3 Level 3: developmental radiotherapy department

In addition to the activities of a level 2 department, efforts will be devoted to more basic radiobiological research and to the design, development and testing of new imaging, treatment planning, treatment delivery and verification techniques.

The types of human resources and/or necessary skills that will be required at the various levels of radiotherapy department will vary, depending on the principal objective. However, at any level of radiotherapy department, the most important component is the personnel. In some instances, for example in a level 1 department, it may be necessary for one staff member to carry out more than one function or provide more than one skill. Sometimes it may be necessary to make co-operative arrangements with other clinical departments or community services (nursing, dietetic or social services) to assure that the necessary function is performed for the patients being treated.

General guidelines showing the human resource requirements for the three levels of radiotherapy departments are given in Table 1.4

Table 1.4 Guidelines for human resource requirements for radiotherapy departments at various levels

Profession or skill	Level 1	Level 2	Level 3
Radiation oncologist – chief of service	One	One	One
Staff radiation oncologist	Should be available (one-man departments are not recommended)	One or more	Three or more
Radiation physicist – chief	This function must be provided	One	One
Staff radiation physicist	–	One or more	Three or more
Dosimetrist (physics technologist)	May be needed	One or more	One or more
Engineer or equipment maintenance specialist	May be needed	One or more	Two or more
Radiotherapy technologist, supervisor	May be needed	Three	Three or more
Staff radiotherapy technologist for treatment machines	Two or more	Three	Three or more
Technologist for diagnostic X-ray, therapy simulator	May be needed	One or more	One or more
Techologist for brachytherapy	May be needed	One or more	One or more
Nurse	One	Two or more	One or more
Social worker	May be needed	One or more	One or more
Dietitian	May be needed	One or more	One or more
Rehabilitation specialist	May be needed	One or more	One or more
Radiobiologist	–	One or more	One or more

and guidelines for equipment and premises are shown in Tables 1.5 and 1.6.

1.3 ORGANIZATION

The detailed organization of radiation oncology services in any specific country, geographical area or institution will depend on the local conditions, including: priority assigned to cancer treatment, available human and material resources (both quantity and quality), perception by medical colleagues of the outcomes achieved, local biases and preferences. The resulting radiation oncology service may range from a small department (within or outside a local hospital) to a large department in an oncology institute. General conditions considered as the minimum acceptable for providing radiation oncology services are:

- a sufficiently large number of cancer patients to be treated to maintain clinical expertise: a generally accepted minimum number is about 300 new cancer patients per year;
- a fully qualified radiation oncologist available on a full-time basis;
- the availability of megavoltage radiotherapy equipment (equipment operating at or above 2 MV, such as a telecobalt teletherapy machine or an accelerator);
- radiation physics and dosimetry support, at least that of a physicist who provides support to several institutions.

Every radiation oncology department will require out-patient facilities (perhaps as many as 80–90% of the cancer patients could be out-patients) as well as access to hospital beds for those patients requiring them. Other facilities or services which must be available are diagnostic imaging, clinical laboratory services, simple surgery, nursing, rehabilitation and social work. Radiation protection services (training, monitoring, guidance) must be provided for the staff, and the patient's safety must be assured regarding mechanical as well as radiological hazards. An example of the organization of a comprehensive radiotherapy department is shown in Figure 1.3 and an example of the circulation of patients within a hospital-based radiotherapy department is shown in Figure 1.4.

From time to time authoritative national and international scientific and professional groups have provided guidelines for staff and facility requirements. Some examples are given below, to provide a general idea of the approximate numbers and the ranges. Values relevant to any specific geographical, socio-economic, and medical care matrix cannot be indiscriminately applied to another context.

Radiation oncologist
- not less than two per radiotherapy department: no one-man radiotherapy departments

Table 1.5 Guidelines for equipment requirements for radiotherapy departments at various levels

Type of equipment	Level 1	Level 2	Level 3
External beam therapy equipment			
Low-voltage (superficial) X-ray	One	One or more	One or more
Cobalt-60 teletherapy or low-energy accelerator (4–6 MV)	One or more	One or more	One or more
Contact therapy X-ray	–	One or more	One or more
Beta-ray applicator	–	One or more	One or more
Medium-energy accelerator (8–20 MV photons + 6–20 MeV electrons)	–	One or more	One or more
High-energy accelerator (5-50 MV photons + 5-50 MeV electrons)	–	–	One or more
Internal therapy equipment			
Manual afterloading using caesium-137	One or more	Possibly	Possibly
Remote, manually operated afterloading using caesium-137	Possibly	Possibly	–
Remote motor-driven afterloading using caesium-137 and iridium-192	–	Possibly	One or more
Equipment for interstitial therapy	Caesium-137 most practical	Full range of equipment and isotopes may be needed	Full range of equipment and isotopes

Radioisotopes used as unsealed sources			
Equipment for measuring activity and dispensing	Not practical	May be needed	Needed
Treatment planning, simulation and verification			
Small personal computer	Useful	–	–
Dedicated mini-computer	Not practical	May be useful	Useful
Diagnostic X-ray machine used as simulator	Most practical	–	–
Radiotherapy simulator (fluoroscopy)	–	One or more	One or more
Shielding block and treatment aids	Pre-fabricated most practical	Necessary	Necessary
Production equipment for shielding block and treatment aids	May be useful	Necessary	Necessary
Radiation measurements, calibration, radiation protection monitoring			
Ionization chamber and electrometer	Needed if physicist on site	One or more	Several
		Motor-driven automatic isodose plotter	Motor-driven automatic isodose plotter
Phantoms	Simple phantoms may be needed		
Radiation protection monitoring	Personnel monitoring + survey meter	Personnel monitoring + survey meter + special individual monitoring	Personnel monitoring + survey meter + special individual monitoring

Table 1.6 Guidelines for premises requirements for radiotherapy departments at various levels

Purpose of room	Level 1	Level 2	Level 3
Reception and administration			
Reception office	Required	Required	Required
Secretary	Could be combined with reception office	Required	Required
Records	Could be combined with reception and secretary's office	Required	Required
Patient waiting	Required	Required	Required
Patient lavatories	Required	Required	Required
Staff lavatories	Required	Required	Required
Storage; cleaning supplies, trolleys, etc.	Required	Required	Required
Consultation and examination			
Patient consultation	Could be combined with examination room	Required	Required
Patient examination	See above	Required	Required
Clean linens	Required	Required	Required
Dirty linens	May combine as part of clean linens room or other storage area	Required	Required
Treatment			
Treatment room: low-energy X-ray	Required	Required	Required
Treatment room(s): cobalt-60 or low-energy accelerator	Required	Required	Required
Treatment room(s): medium- or high-energy accelerators	Not recommended	Required	Required

Sealed sources storage	Required	Possibly	Possibly
Remote afterloading machine, manually operated	Could be combined with sealed sources storage	Possibly	Possibly
Remote afterloading machine, motor driven	Not recommended	Possibly	Required
Unsealed sources treatment room	Not recommended	Required	Required
Radioactive waste storage	Not recommended	Required	Required
Laboratory/treatment planning			
Mould room and assembly of devices	Only if critical assessment shows it is needed	Required	Required
Physics and dosimetry including computation equipment	Only if critical assessment shows it is needed	Required	Required
Workshop, electronic and mechanical fabrication	Not recommended	Possibly	Required
Diagnostic X-ray simulator	Simple radiography	Image-intensified fluoroscopy	Image-intensified fluoroscopy
Staff conference/treatment planning/records review	Possibly	Required	Required
Staff rooms			
Radiation oncologist(s)	At least one office	As required	As required
Physicist	At least one office	As required	As required
Radiotherapy technologists (radiographers)	At least one office	As required	As required
Hospital facilities			
Operating room	Access to a hospital operating room	Access to a hospital or possibly a room in the radiotherapy department	A room in the radiotherapy department may be needed
Hospital beds	Access to hospital beds	Access to hospital beds	Access to hospital beds

- one additional staff radiation oncologist for each 200–250 patients treated annually

Radiation physicist
- one physicist per centre (minimum)
- one additional physicist for each 400 patients treated annually

Radiotherapy technologist
- one technologist for low-voltage radiograph and sealed sources
- a minimum of three trained technologists per department

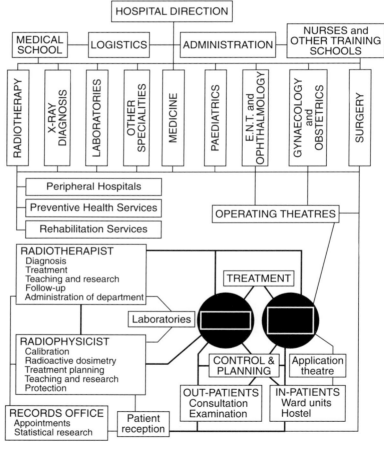

Figure 1.3 Example of the organization of a comprehensive cancer centre.

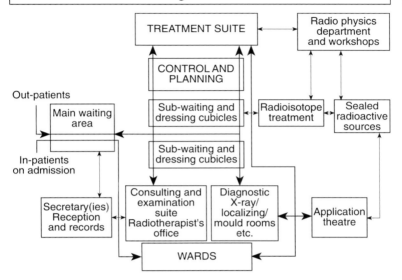

Figure 1.4 Example of the circulation of patients in a radiotherapy department.

- two or three per megavoltage unit if up to 40 patients treated daily per unit
- four to six per megavoltage unit if up to 60 patients treated daily per unit

The assumptions upon which any such guideline values are based must be understood and thoroughly analysed before use. To assist in understanding the basis for guidelines an example is provided for the estimated number of cancer patients that can be treated and the population coverage by one megavoltage teletherapy machine. It can be appreciated that changes in the assumptions could easily result in quite different values.

1. The first assumption is that six patients (including those treated for both palliative and curative intent) can be treated in one hour.
2. It is then assumed that the working schedule is 8 hours per day, 5 days per week, for 50 weeks per year.

   6 treatments/h × 8 h/day × 5 days/week × 50 weeks/year = 12 000 treatments year.

3. Assume:
   (a) 40% of treatments are for cure with 32 fractions (average) of 200 cGy per fraction.
   (b) 60% of treatments are for palliation with 12 fractions (average) of 200 cGy per fraction

   $40\% \times 12\,000 = 4800$ treaments: at   32 fractions/patient
   $= 150$ patients/year
   $60\% \times 12\,000 = 7200$ treaments: at   12 fractions/patient
   $= 600$ patients/year
   Therefore, the total number of patients that can be treated is 750 per year.

4. Assume that the cancer incidence is 140 cases per 100 000 population and that 40% of new cancer patients will be treated with radiotherapy.

$$\frac{750 \text{ patients}}{\text{year}} \times \frac{100\,000}{140} \times \frac{1}{40\%} = 1.3 \text{ million}$$

Therefore, the population that could be served by one megavoltage unit is 1.3 million.

In many actual situations the assumptions listed above must be adjusted because of the complexity of treatment, the output of the radiation source (for example, it may not be possible to maintain a dose of 200 cGy per treatment as a telecobalt source decays or it may not be possible to maintain an hourly throughput of six patients), breakdowns of complex electrical equipment, and the possibility of treating patients for palliation using less than an average of 12 fractions per patient. The amount and complexity of treatment simulation, quality, assurance and treatment delivery verification procedures will also influence estimates, as will the health status of the patient and the corresponding ability to co-operate during treatment.

2

Clinical fundamentals

2.1 INTRODUCTION

It has been estimated that if the best available (optimum) method of treatment were used, then one-third of all cancers could be cured. The majority of cancer patients are treated with surgery alone or in combination with radiotherapy and/or chemotherapy (60%), about 30% with radiotherapy, and about 10% with chemotherapy. Radiotherapy also has an important role in palliation. In some developed countries, up to 60% of all cancer patients are either treated for cure or for palliation with radiotherapy.

Ideally all patients should be treated in centres that have the necessary resources in terms of specialized medical and non-medical staff as well as the appropriate equipment. Patients for whom cure is possible would have a much better chance of successful treatment if all the facilities for a correct diagnosis and optimum treatment were used for their benefit. This is especially important when considering that the best chance for cure is through the right treatment the first time. Even when cure is not expected, no patient should be deprived of the possibility to have painful or discomforting symptoms palliated.

Depending on the extent of the disease, and with the patient's situation and interest in view, the best type of treatment (even including the possibility of no specific treatment if its effect would worsen the patient's condition) should, ideally, be determined by an oncological team. Figure 2.1 illustrates the functional oncological aspects that should be considered for the optimal planning of the treatment and the subsequent management of the cancer patient. In some places where a certain specialist is not available, it may be necessary to rely more heavily on the other team members.

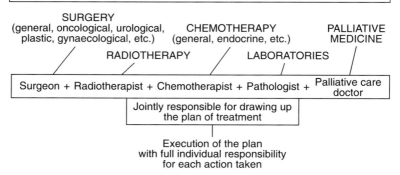

Figure 2.1 Teamwork in the planning of cancer treatment and the management of patients.

The objective of the team approach is to ensure that the modality for cancer treatment is not decided by only one specialist or only considering one modality. The desired result of the team approach is to choose the optimum treatment or combination of treatments which will be of most benefit to the patient, including considerations of the least discomfort and the best quality of life following the treatment.

The modalities which should be considered, as a single treatment method or in combination with others, are radiotherapy, surgery and chemotherapy (including hormone therapy) and palliative care. Based on experience accumulated over many years, certain modalities have emerged as the treatment of choice for specific types and stages of cancers, while for other cancers the optimum choice may be a combination of more than one modality or may depend on the level of expertise available locally in the treating institution. Certainly, as stated in WHO TRS No. 322, Cancer Treatment, 'Good surgery is preferable to bad radiotherapy but, equally, good radiotherapy is preferable to bad surgery'. Palliative care alone is often the most relevant approach.

Examples of modalities for which a general agreement has emerged based on current knowledge are:

Radiotherapy, principally for curative intent (radical treatment):

- breast
- mouth and lip, pharynx, larynx (head and neck)

- female genital organs
- skin
- lymphomas
- primary brain tumours
- prostate
- unresectable sarcomas

Radiotherapy, principally for palliative intent:

- bony or intracranial metastases
- control of chronic bleeding
- oesophagus
- lung
- reduction of elevated intracranial pressure

Surgery, principally for curative intent (radical treatment):

- colon and rectum
- bladder
- breast
- female genital organs
- lung
- skin
- stomach
- prostate

Surgery, principally for palliative intent:

- amputation of extremities
- resection of infected, bleeding or obstructive cancers
- severance of sensory nerve tracts
- stomach, colon, rectum
- lung, liver, pancreas, oesophagus

Chemotherapy, principally for curative intent (radical treatment):

- choriocarcinoma
- leukaemias and lymphomas
- testes
- paediatric malignancies

Chemotherapy, principally for palliative intent:

- breast
- brain

Table 2.1 Initial treatment by various modalities and combinations[a]

Site (ICD-9 Code No.)	Total registrations for this site	Percentage of patients registered during the period 1982–1984 according to modality of treatment							
		S alone	R alone	C alone	S + R	S + C	R + C	S + R + C	Untreated
Stomach (151)	5 626	46	1	3	1.5	6	0.5	1	41
Colon (153)	6 932	72.5	0.4	1	3	5	0.1	1	17
Rectum and anus (154)	3 980	63.5	3	1	12	3	0.5	3	14
Pancreas (157)	2 904	44	1	2.5	1	6	0.5	2	43
Trachea, bronchus and lung (162)	17 627	11	19	11	4	2	10	2	41
Skin tumours (not including malignant melanoma) (173)	10 791	48	39	0.5	8.5	0.2	0.2	0.3	3
Female breast (174)	11 822	21.3	5.5	10	25	11.5	7	14.5	5
Cervix uteri (invasive) (180)	1 565	18	36	1	26	1	5	4	9
Body of uterus (182)	1 888	18	5	2.5	23	14	4	26	7.5
Prostate (185)	4 968	36	3	12	12	17	3	8	9
Bladder (188)	4 656	53	7.5	0.5	22.5	4	1	3	8.5
Hodgkin's disease (201)	678	4.2	14.2	26	13.5	14	12	8	8
Lymphoid leukaemia (204)	825	4.3	3	26.5	0.2	13	6	8	39
All sites (104–234)	102 992	34.6	12.4	6.7	10.4	7	4.2	5.2	19.5

[a]Based on data obtained from the Thames Cancer registry, Statistical Report on Cancer Registrations in the SC and SW Thames Regional Health Authority Areas, 1982–1984. compilation by Radiation Medicine Unit, World Health Organization, September 1991.
S = Surgery, R = Radiotherapy, C = Chemotherapy.

- leukaemias and lymphomas
- prostate

The experience for common cancer sites in an area with a population-based cancer registry and well-developed treatment services is shown in Table 2.1.

In some cases there is no clear preference, for example in early breast cancer and early cancer of the cervix (i.e. cervical cancer that has progressed beyond the *in situ* stage). The optimum treatment for any single patient should be decided by the oncological team after consideration of the available treatment modalities and expertise, as well as the physical status and the preference of the informed patient.

Before deciding on the appropriate treatment the oncologist must carefully assess the patient's general condition and type and stage of tumour. Many patients over 70 years or with coincident diseases such as diabetes, hypertension or chronic cardiac and pulmonary conditions may be unable to tolerate radical treatment. Other patients may require parenteral nutrition or transfusion before radiotherapy.

The extent of tumour should be assessed and classified in the TNM system (UICC, 1987) by thorough clinical examination and appropriate surgical, medical, haematological and radiological investigations. The site, size, mobility and stage of the tumour should be carefully recorded, as should the presence of local invasion, e.g. of bone and muscle, or distant metastases. Lymph node involvement should be recorded including size and mobility. Most tumours in stages 1, 2 and 3 may be suitable for radical treatment if the patient's condition is good, while most stage 4 tumours will require palliative treatment only.

The oncologist must next decide whether to offer the patient radical or palliative treatment or to provide supportive care only, i.e. no anti-neoplastic modality.

2.2 TREATMENT POLICY

2.2.1 Radical radiotherapy

Radical radiotherapy is used for patients in good general condition and with limited tumours where there is a reasonable chance of cure. The dose will be high, e.g. 60–66 Gy/30–33 fr/6–6½ weeks and some side-effects of the treatment are inevitable, e.g. diarrhoea and dysuria in the radical radiotherapy of cervical carcinoma. These can be controlled by drugs and are acceptable if the disease can be cured.

Radical radiotherapy may be used as sole treatment in early lymphoma, solitary plasmacytoma, carcinoma of the cervix, vagina, nasopharynx, early carcinomas of the head and neck, skin, lip, bladder, prostate, oesophagus and penis. These are all either highly radiosensitive tumours (lymphoma, plasmacytoma) or situations in which experience has shown that radiotherapy alone has a reasonable cure rate. In early larynx cancer, cure rates are marginally higher with surgery but radiotherapy preserves the voice; the policy is therefore to use radiotherapy first and save surgery for salvage.

Alternatively, it may be used in conjunction with chemotherapy, as generally in lymphoma stages III and IV, myeloma, some testicular tumours, Ewing's sarcoma, lymphoma of bone, early paediatric solid tumours, endemic Kaposi's sarcoma, carcinomas of the anus and anal canal, cerebral radiotherapy in acute lymphatic leukaemia, small-cell lung cancer. In many of these tumours, chemotherapy is the principal modality of treatment but radiotherapy is needed either to deal with residual tumour or, as in acute lymphocytic leukaemia, to cope with 'sanctuary sites', such as the meninges, where the drugs fail to reach.

Post-operative radiotherapy (occasionally pre-operative) is usually given in carcinoma of the breast, oesophagus, thyroid, uterus, Fallopian tubes, vulva, ovary, kidney, bladder, other genito-urinary sites, skin and lip, biliary tract, more advanced head and neck cancers, salivary gland tumours, paediatric solid tumours, soft tissue sarcomas, gliomas and other brain tumours, orbital tumours, colorectal cancer, endocrine tumours and melanoma.

Although many of the above are not radiosensitive, radiotherapy can devitalize microscopic disease left behind after surgery. Conservation surgery is being increasingly practised today, especially for cancer of the breast, salivary glands and rectum, and requires radical post-operative radiotherapy. Decisions regarding conservation surgery and radiotherapy should be made jointly in advance.

2.2.2 Palliative radiotherapy

Palliative radiotherapy is given when it is recognized that the patient is beyond cure, but nevertheless suffers from some symptom or symptoms which radiotherapy can alleviate.

(a) Pain

Bone pain from metastases of breast, bronchus or prostate or from myeloma responds well to short-term radiotherapy. The headache resulting from cerebral metastases from carcinoma or leukaemia also responds well; headaches from direct invasion of bone, e.g. from nasopharyngeal carcinoma, respond less well. Pain from liver metastases is best treated by other methods, e.g. steroids. Pain from nerve root infiltration responds unpredictably to radiotherapy – if anaesthetic procedures are available they should be tried.

(b) Obstruction

Malignancies cause visceral obstruction in many situations which may be relieved by radiotherapy. Oesophageal obstruction, lung atelectasis or superior vena caval obstruction from bronchial carcinoma, ureteric obstruction from carcinoma of the cervix or bladder, and lymphoma of the stomach causing outlet obstruction often benefit from palliative radiotherapy. Lymphoedema of the upper or lower limb caused by axillary lymphadenopathy from cervical cancer is only partially relieved, commonly because of a superimposed venous thrombosis.

(c) Bleeding

Bleeding causes great anxiety and is common in advanced cancers of the cervix, uterus, bladder, pharynx, bronchus or oral cavity. Palliative radiotherapy is of great value in all of these. Haematuria from hypernephroma is best treated by nephrectomy.

(d) Ulceration

Ulceration of the chest wall in breast carcinoma or of the perineum in rectal carcinoma – sure signs of incurable disease – cause great distress. Radiotherapy can relieve the ulceration, pain and foul odour, and so improve quality of life.

(e) Pathological fracture

Radiotherapy to a large deposit in a weight-bearing bone, whether secondary to carcinoma or primary as in Ewing's sarcoma or myeloma, may prevent fracture. Once a fracture has occurred, radiotherapy should be preceded by fixation of the affected bone, so that the patient may be kept as mobile as possible. In some circumstances, internal fixation should precede radiotherapy in order to obviate an impending fracture.

(f) Relief of neurological deficits

Retrobulbar tumours or choroidal metastases secondary to breast carcinoma regress with radiotherapy, which usually preserves vision. Paraparesis from spinal cord compression may improve with radiotherapy especially if of short history (less than 24 hours) and resulting from radiosensitive tumours, but in most situations radiotherapy should be preceded by surgical decompression.

(g) Relief of systemic symptoms

Non-metastatic effects of small-cell lung carcinoma, e.g. neuropathy or myopathy, are reduced by radiotherapy to the primary tumour. Myasthenia gravis associated with thymic neoplasia responds well to thymic radiotherapy. Night sweats, fever or weight loss may improve with palliative radiotherapy to large lymphomatous masses.

Since the patient's life expectancy may be short, the overall time for palliative radiotherapy should also be short. Typical regimes are 10 Gy single fraction, 25 Gy in five fractions or 30 Gy in ten fractions (depending on the field size). As far as possible, palliative radiotherapy should be designed so as not to cause side-effects.

2.3 CAUSES OF SUCCESS OR FAILURE OF RADIOTHERAPY

2.3.1 Tumour factors

(a) Radiosensitivity

Radiosensitivity is an inherent property of the tumour cells. Tumours vary in radiosensitivity and some are listed below in descending order of radiosensitivity:

- seminoma
- lymphocytic lymphoma
- other lymphomas, leukaemia, myeloma
- some embryonal sarcomas, small-cell lung cancer, choriocarcinoma
- Ewing's sarcoma
- squamous cell carcinoma:
    poorly differentiated
    well differentiated
- adenocarcinoma of breast, rectum
- transitional cell carcinoma
- hepatoma
- melanoma
- glioma, other sarcomas

Seminoma and lymphoma are the most radiosensitive. Choriocarcinoma is highly sensitive but generally treated by chemotherapy.
Melanomas are generally resistant to conventional radiotherapy due
to their wide 'shoulder' on the cell survival curve, but good
response rates are obtained with high-dose-per-fraction radiotherapy
regimens (e.g. 30 Gy/6 fr/3 weeks). Glioma and adult soft-tissue
sarcoma are radioresistant but radiotherapy is still of value post-
operatively for microscopic disease.

(b) Tumour volume

Radiation can eradicate small tumours more easily than large
tumours (large tumours have more cells, also a higher proportion of
hypoxic cells and non-cycling (G_0) cells, which are less radiosensitive). A regimen of 50 Gy in 5 weeks can usually eradicate
occult squamous carcinoma in neck or groin nodes or occult breast
carcinoma in axillary nodes, but palpable nodal disease requires full
dosage.

(c) Tumour site

The curability of a tumour depends also on the dose permissible to
the adjacent normal tissues, since they are inevitably included in the
radiation field. The high cure rate of early cervical carcinoma owes

much to the remarkable tolerance to radiation of the vaginal mucosa.

2.3.2 Normal tissue factors

An understanding of how radiation can affect normal tissues is crucial to the safe practice of radiotherapy. The most sensitive organs are the bone marrow, gonads, gut mucosa, lymphatic tissue and the lens of the eye. Liver, kidney, lung, skin, breast, gut wall and nervous tissue are moderately sensitive, while bone, connective tissue and muscle are relatively insensitive.

(a) Highly radiosensitive tissues

Haemopoietic tissues
The bone marrow is exceedingly sensitive to radiation and a single whole-body dose of 4 Gy would cause lethal myelosuppression in about 50% of patients. Allogeneic bone marrow transplantation has permitted total-body irradiation to higher doses (e.g. 10 Gy) as part of the therapy for acute leukaemia, and other malignances.

Gonads
The testes and ovaries are highly sensitive to radiation. In the testes doses as low as 100 cGy can cause marked oligospermia, which may be permanent after 200 cGy. In the ovary, doses of 10–12 Gy will cause amenorrhoea in most patients, the proportion being higher in older women. Secondary sex characteristics are also affected in women, but not in men since the androgen-producing Leydig cells are more radioresistant.

(b) Moderately radiosensitive tissues

Gastrointestinal tract
All parts of the alimentary tract are moderately radiosensitive, especially crypt cells of the small intestine. Thus radiotherapy for intra-abdominal malignancy is limited by gastrointestinal side-effects. The acute effects are nausea, vomiting and diarrhoea. Late effects after radical dosage include malabsorption, rectal ulceration, bleeding, stricture or fistula. The rectal dose is the limiting factor in pelvic radiotherapy for cervical carcinoma.

Skin

As the skin dose increases, erythema and first dry and then moist desquamation, epilation and loss of sebaceous and sweat gland function follow radiation. Other effects include pigmentation (or depigmentation), fibrosis, subcutaneous atrophy and telangiectasia.

Nervous tissue

Brain and spinal cord tolerance are both around 50 Gy with conventional fractionation (180–200 cGy daily) but tolerance is reduced with large fractions or concomitant chemotherapy. Hypothalamus, brain stem, optic chiasm and lumbar or cervical cord are often thought to be more sensitive to radiation. Radiation myelitis is a tragic complication of radiotherapy, with hemi- or paraplegia, sensory signs, Brown-Séquard syndrome and sphincter dysfunction. Consequently most clinicians are rightly very cautious about spinal cord dose and do not exceed 40–45 Gy for a 10 cm cord length. Hypertension can increase cord radiosensitivity. Lhermitte's sign (parasthesia in the extremities on neck flexion) is a self-limiting condition, associated with arachnoiditis, without serious long-term consequences.

The eye

The principal radiosensitive structures in the orbit are the lens, the lacrimal gland and the lashes. Cataract has followed doses of 200 cGy although it is doubtful whether many vision impairing cataracts have been caused by total doses less than 20 Gy. The lacrimal gland has comparable sensitivity to that of sweat glands. The tolerance of eye lashes is about 23–28 Gy. Thus the main hazards of radiation to the eye at doses of 30–40 Gy are cataract, a dry eye and loss of the protective reflex.

Lung

Radiation pneumonitis is a clinical syndrome which may follow 1–3 months after radiation involving the lungs, e.g. for breast, lung or oesophageal carcinoma or in total-body irradiation for acute myelogenous leukaemia. There is sloughing of alveolar cells, endothelial damage and alveolo-capillary block. Symptoms include cough, dyspnoea, cyanosis, fever and night sweats, and, three to six months later, pulmonary fibrosis. Steroids help in the acute phase. The threshold for pneumonitis is 7–8 Gy in a single fraction or 20 Gy/ 10 fr.

Kidney

Doses of 23–25 Gy over 3–5 weeks to the kidney can cause acute radiation nephritis or chronic radiation nephropathy (within months to years) with proteinuria, anaemia, hypertension and uraemia. Renal tolerance is lower in children.

Liver

Liver tolerance is 30 Gy/15 fr in 3 weeks and 75% of patients will suffer from liver dysfunction after 40 Gy in 4 weeks. Tolerance is reduced after chemotherapy.

(c) Less radiosensitive tissue

Bone growth may be affected following radiotherapy in children, especially where the epiphyseal plate received high dosage. Radiotherapy to vertebrae may cause stunting and kyphoscoliosis. Avascular necrosis of the head of the humerus or femur may occur in adults following radical dosage.

2.3.3 Other late sequelae of radiation

Three other potential major late effects of radiation include carcinogenesis, teratogenesis and mutagenesis.

(a) Carcinogenesis

Historical evidence shows that radiation can predispose to the development of malignancy. Survivors of atomic bomb explosions have had an increased risk of neoplasms, especially leukaemias. Uranium miners who inhaled radon gas, the early radiologists, children irradiated for ringworm, and patients given radium injections for tuberculosis have all shown an increase in malignancies of lung, skin, thyroid and bone respectively. There is a latent interval (under 10 years for leukaemia, 10–20 years for solid tumours). The risk is higher when chemotherapy is also used.

(b) Teratogenesis

Irradiation of the pregnant woman is contra-indicated. In the first trimester the major risks are fetal resorption or malformations – these are not specific for radiation but the incidence is increased over that expected. Later in pregnancy, growth retardation and mental subnormality may occur.

(c) Mutagenesis

This refers to alteration of the genetic material of somatic or germ cells due to irradiation. In the somatic cell the main risk is carcinogenesis as above. In the germ cells mutation leads to fetal death or subnormality, but in humans it is thought that most germ cell mutations are not viable. This is why reports of abnormalities in children born to fathers who underwent testicular irradiation are rare.

2.4 TREATMENT PLANNING

2.4.1 Optimization

The practice of radiotherapy, like all other medical treatment, has the goal of curing disease and sparing normal tissues. However, in the treatment of cancer the therapeutic ratio, i.e. effect on tumour/ effect on normal tissue, is not large. Cancer cells also closely resemble their normal counterparts and the treatment modalities available – surgery, radiotherapy and chemotherapy – are relatively non-specific as compared to, for example, penicillin in the treatment of pneumonia. Thus extreme care must be taken to ensure that the treatment is optimum in order to gain the small advantage of destroying tumour over damaging tissues. Since the dose–response curves for radiation effect are very steep, the first goal is to deliver a homogeneous dose into the volume to be treated. Since tumours rarely solely occupy a compact volume but rather infiltrate normal tissues, this concept of homogeneity of dose must be respected. If even one small portion of a tumour is significantly underdosed the treatment will fail; on the other hand if a small portion of the treated volume containing a normal tissue is significantly overdosed, a treatment complication may result (Figure 2.2).

The clinician usually assigns a higher merit value to cure rather than complication, but this may often be difficult: a serious debilitating chronic complication, for example recurrent intestinal obstructions and perforation or transverse myelitis, may be considered a fate worse than rapid death from a tumour.

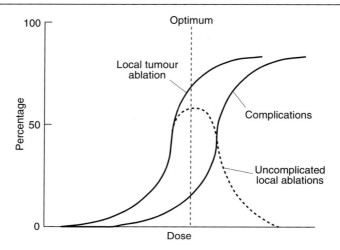

Figure 2.2 Diagram showing how local tumour ablation and complications rise with dose. By subtracting complications from local tumour ablations, a bell-shaped curve is obtained, showing uncomplicated local ablations that are the optimum results for a particular dose range.

Therefore, the challenge is to design radiotherapy treatments, using all one's clinical knowledge and experience, so that the best possibility of tumour cure can be achieved without a significant risk of serious complications. The factors in planning include the volume to be treated, and the dosage to be given.

2.4.2 Volume

It is clearly established that tolerance to radiation diminishes as the treatment volume increases. The therapeutic goal must be to treat as small a volume as possible, yet adequate enough to treat every tumour cell. Thus five different types of volumes have been defined (Figure 2.3). The gross tumour volume (GTV) denotes the demonstrated tumour. The clinical target volume (CTV) denotes the demonstrated tumour (when present) and also volumes with suspected (subclinical) tumour (e.g. margin around the GTV, and regional lymph nodes, that are considered to need treatment). The CTV is thus a *pure anatomic clinical concept*. The planning target volume (PTV) consists of the CTV(s) and a margin to account for variation in size, shape, and position relative to the treatment beam(s). The PTV is thus a *geometric concept*, used to ensure that the CTV receives the prescribed dose, and it is (like the patient/ tissues concerned) defined *in relation to a fixed coordinate* system. In Figure 2.3 the magnitude of foreseen movements by the patient may change the CTV in different directions. Treated volume is the volume that receives a dose that is considered significant for local cure or palliation, and irradiated volume is the volume that receives a dose that is considered significant for normal tissue tolerance (other than those specifically defined for organs at risk).

(a) Limiting normal tissue volumes

The mirror reflection of cure in optimization is conservation of normal tissue structure and function. The first principle of medicine espoused by Galen was *'Primum non nocere'* ('First, do no harm'). In order to obey this principle, yet achieve the goal of cure, the radiation oncologist must know the factors leading to damage of tissue by radiation. These include volume and dosage. Thus, in addition to the concept of target volume, treatment planning must include some method of defining dose–volume limitations in the

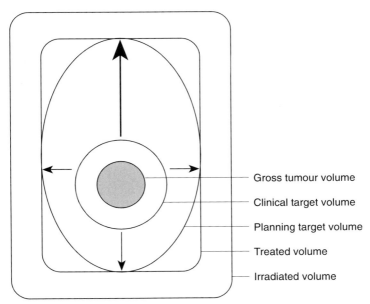

Figure 2.3 Schematic illustration of the different volumes to be considered in radiation therapy: from ICRU Report No. 50.

volume outside the target, i.e, the region exposed to radiation. It is already assumed that the dose to be delivered to the target volume is limited by the tolerance of normal tissues. Otherwise an infinitely large dose could be delivered in order to achieve complete tumour destruction. In practice, the limitations of dosage and volume can be set by the construction of one or more 'limiting isodose' contours. For the advantage of the physicist/treatment planning dosimetrist, these isodose contours can be defined by values corresponding to the percentage of the maximum dose, e.g. < 0.6 (less than 60% of the maximum dose), while the target volume dose may be defined as, e.g. > 0.9 (more than 90% of the maximum dose).

(b) 'Shrinking' volumes

Modern radiobiology allows us to estimate the radiation doses needed to sterilize cells. Knowing that micrometastases involve smaller numbers of cells, more sophisticated tailoring of the treatment to the clinical problem can be done. Since a solid tumour invades and spreads by sending out small numbers of cells into adjacent tissues one can conceive of more than one target volume at different dose levels. In practice, this involves the initial definition of a larger target volume which, after a certain dose is given, is reduced to a smaller volume, often corresponding closely to the previously defined tumour volume. This concept accomplishes two things: it permits a larger than usual treatment volume to be used, knowing that tissue tolerance will be preserved because of the lower dose to that volume, and it permits a higher dose than usual to the second or 'cone-down' volume which will encompass the more radioresistant solid central tumour (Figure 2.4).

In fact, a variety of combinations can be imagined: normal dose/ normal volume followed by high dose/small volume or low dose/ large volume followed by high dose/small volume, etc. This is now often referred to as the 'field within the field' technique.

The fundamental advantage of this concept is to preserve normal tissue tolerance and still allow more effective dosage to radioresistant tumours. Its practical application requires an even higher level of co-operation between clinician, treatment planner and therapy technician than usual and the risk of increased error in treatment must be carefully considered before embarking on this approach.

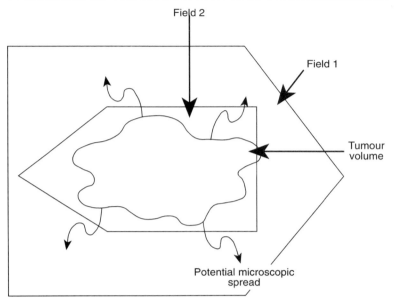

Figure 2.4 'Field within a field' technique. Field 1 is intended to treat gross disease plus microscopic extension. Field 2 is intended to treat gross (bulk) disease only. Various combinations are possible based on clinical judgement and objective clinical findings (X-ray, pathology, etc.).

2.4.3 Dosage

The term *dosage* includes all the factors in delivering radiation to a specific point or volume in the patient. These factors include the dose per fraction, the number of fractions, the overall time of treatment, and the structure of fractions within the overall time, for example, 'split-course' treatment. In cases of brachytherapy, a very important additional factor is dose rate, with significantly different clinical responses per unit dose occurring following high dose rates of the order of 10–100 cGy/min as compared to a low dose rate of the order of 0.1 to 1.0 cGy/min with a spectrum of responses throughout this range. Dosage schedules are as follows:

- 'Normal' fractionation: 4–6 daily fractions per week: overall time, 3–6 weeks;
- Hypofractionation: less than four daily fractions per week;
- Hyperfractionation: two or more fractions per day (of reduced size) with overall time similar to normal fractionation;

- Accelerated hyperfractionation: two or more fractions per day (of 'normal' size) with reduced overall time;
- Split-course schedule: generally two abbreviated courses of normal fractionation separated by 1 or 2 weeks of rest.

For purposes of this basic introduction to treatment planning only normal fractionation is discussed in any detail.

(a) Tumour lethal dose

As previously mentioned, it can be assumed that an infinitely large dose can cure any cancer. However, we are ultimately limited by normal tissue tolerance. Thus, there has developed, by practical experience, a concept of 'tumour dose' which in reality reflects the limits imposed by normal tissue and expresses the best possible dose schedule. Thus typical tumour doses for carcinoma are 60 Gy in 30 fractions over 6 weeks (popular in the USA) or 50 Gy in 15 fractions over 3 weeks (the Manchester schedule). Yet, from clinical experience and radiobiological assumptions, the dose needed to cure 100% of very small cancers is considerably less while the probability of cure with these dose schedules rapidly diminishes when tumour volumes exceed $100 \, cm^3$. In addition to numerous other criticisms, the use of empirical equations to calculate tumour dose schedules is seriously limited by this fact. However, since so much has been published using the NSD concept and its corollary, the TDF system, it is important to be familiar with the essential manipulations. The TDF value of 100 is equivalent to the dose value of both the American and Manchester schedules quoted above. Thus (from Table 14-5 of Hall's text; Hall, 1994) 260 cGy/fraction $\times$ 20 fractions (5 fractions per week) = 52 Gy in 4 weeks (TDF 99). From practical experience it appears that this or the very similar schedule 50 Gy in 4 weeks (TDF = 93) can cure a majority of superficial (T1) buccal mucosa carcinomas without a serious late morbidity. However, the probability of cure of a T3 carcinoma with this dose is probably low. Thus a TDF of 110 or 120 may be necessary, provided that the normal tissue tolerances are respected. On the other hand, Hodgkin's disease and other lymphomas can be locally cured with TDF values of about 70, and seminomas with TDF of 50. It has been demonstrated that the cure of microscopic carcinoma (such as in N0 lymphatics) can be accomplished with high probability with TDF values of 80. Table 2.2 lists typical doses

Table 2.2 Doses required to give estimated 90% probability of local tumour control

Tumour type	Stage or volume	Dosage range (Gy/weeks)	TDF
Carcinoma,	N0 (subclinical)	50/5	82
adeno and	T1	50/4	93
squamous	Early T2	52/4	100
		60/6	
	T2–T3, N1	70/7	115
		66/6	
		57/4	
	Early T4, N3	73.50/7	
	< 20 cm^3	70/6	125
		60/4	
	> 20 cm^3	> 80/8	> 132
Lymphoma	< 100 cm^3	30/3	50
Hodgkin's	> 100 cm^3	40/4	66
Lymphosarcoma	< 100 cm^3	30/3	50
Histiocytic	< 200 cm^3	45/4.5	75
lymphoma			
Seminoma	N1–N3	30/3	60
Plasmacytoma	< 100 cm^3	35/3.5	60
Sarcomas	T2–T3	> 70/6	> 125

needed. These TDF values are valid for overall times between 3 and 6 weeks using the table for five fractions/week.

(b) Tolerance dose

Just as we attempt to estimate the probability of cure with specific doses, it is important to estimate the probability of complications. In contrast to tumour cure, as previously discussed, the dose to produce a complication becomes less as the volume of irradiated normal tissue increases. Thus an estimate of complication probability should include some geometric value, i.e. volume, area (for the skin) or length (for the spinal cord), as well as dose. In practice, one or more treatment planning contours are taken in the region of interest. The target volume and critical normal organs or tissues (kidney, cord, gut or lung, for example) are also traced. Then using data from Table 2.3, the clinician traces isodose contours with limiting doses in terms of percentage maximum dose.

Table 2.3 Tolerance doses (estimated to give 5% probability of significant tissue damage)

Tissue	Dimension	Dosage (Gy/ weeks)	TDF
Connective tissue	< 500 cm^3	63/6	107
	> 500 cm^3	60/6	100
Liver	Whole organ	30/3	50
	< 50% of organ	40/4	66
Kidney	Whole organ	20/2	33
	< 1/3 of organ	60/6	100
Lung	Whole organ	30/3	50
	< 100 cm^3	60/6	100
Skin	< 2 cm (diameter)	90/3	200
	< 10 cm (diameter)	55/3	125
	< 30 cm (diameter)	45/3	92
Spinal cord	< 5 cm (length)	45/3	92
	< 10 cm	50/5	82
	> 10 cm	45/4.5	75
Intestine	< 100 cm^3	45/4.5	75
	Whole abdomen	30/3	50

2.4.4 Optimization procedure

The treatment planner should optimize the treatment by giving the highest and most homogeneous dose contributions to the target volume, the lowest possible dose contributions to the organs at risk outside the target volume, and the highest possible ratio of integral dose contributions in the target volume to integral dose to tissues outside this volume. In practice, without a treatment planning computer, this is accomplished by selecting one or more beams with sizes matched to the target volume and arranging them, by trial and error, but also with intuition and experience, so that these aims are best achieved.

- A good plan is usually a simple plan with as few fields as will serve the purpose.
- The patient treatment position (in which the contours are obtained) should be as comfortable as possible and reproducible.
- For a given beam, the most efficient path is through the nearest surface; for telecobalt, any path longer than 12 cm is relatively inefficient.

- Isocentric techniques are easy to set up but an indiscriminate number of beams can be inefficient.
- Three fields, non-opposing, are desirable but require accurate contours, localization and verification, which are still a problem in many radiotherapy departments.

This process of optimization involves the treatment planner and the clinician in a collaborative effort. There will be frequent instances where the required constraints cannot be fulfilled. The clinician must be prepared to make compromises in order to achieve optimum conditions of treatment.

2.4.5 Field arrangements

For single-field treatments, an applied dose is used where the radiotherapist wishes to prescribe the dose on the skin surface, or a depth dose where the dose must be given at a certain depth. With megavoltage beams, the maximum dose is not delivered to the skin but at a level below the skin which increases with increasing beam energy (Table 2.4). If the radiotherapist wishes to ensure that part or all of the surface receives the maximum dose, then it is necessary to apply bolus, i.e tissue-equivalent, material (wax or wet gauze) of a thickness equivalent to the build-up depth for the energy of radiation, e.g. 0.5 cm for telecobalt, 1.2 cm for 6 MV linear accelerator.

Table 2.4 Depths at which dose is 100%, 80% and 50% of maximum dose for some common photon energies

Photon beam energy	Depth (cm) for percentages of maximum dose		
	100%	80%	50%
230 kV	0	3.0	6.8
Co60	0.5	4.7	11.6
4 MV	1.0	5.6	13.0
6 MV	1.2	6.8	15.6
10 MV	2.0	7.8	19.0
25 MV	3.0	10.2	21.8

Central axis data for 10 cm × 10 cm beam for 230 dV (2 mm Cu half-value layer) at 50 cm SSD, Co 60 and 4 MV at 80 cm SSD and 6 MV, 10 MV and 25 MV at 100 cm SSD.

This is commonly done where scars need to be treated or tumour involves skin or is close to the surface.

Parallel opposing plain fields are suitable for many clinical situations, e.g. in pelvis, abdomen, head and neck. Where the body contour is not uniform throughout the field, wedges may be necessary as tissue compensation. Parallel unwedged fields are normally used with equal weighting, but for lesions not in the midline (e.g. in brain) 2:1 or 3:1 weighting may be used (from the affected side). Most paired field arrangements other than parallel fields will employ the use of wedges. Wedges help to restore dose homogeneity. A wedge angles the dose distribution of the beam, e.g. a 45° wedge in a telecobalt unit angles the 50% isodose through 45°. Wedge fields are commonly arranged such that the angle between the beams (hinge angle) is related to the wedge angle by the equation: wedge angle × 2 = hinge angle.

Three- or four-field plans are commonly used for deep tumours, e.g. oesophagus, bladder, prostate, cervix. Higher energy beams have greater skin sparing, better dose at depth, sharper penumbra and greater bone sparing than telecobalt. These are all advantageous in the treatment of deep-seated tumours as long as the characteristics of the beam in the particular clinical situation are clearly understood. In parallel opposing fields with separations of 18 cm or more, e.g. in obese persons or in lateral pelvic fields, telecobalt gives too low a dose at the midplane. On the other hand, the higher energy machine is not superior in all clinical situations. For whole-brain treatment, with parallel opposing fields, telecobalt gives a superior distribution compared with a 25 MV linear accelerator.

Rotation therapy is an infinite multiple-field technique. It is best suited to fields which are less than 10 cm in width and for centrally located lesions such as those in prostate, bladder, cervix and oesophagus. However, compared with multiple-field techniques, rotation therapy gives a less sharp edge to treatment volume and larger volumes of normal tissues are irradiated.

Electron beams are described in Chapter 1. Their clinical significance lies in the sharp cut-off of dose at a depth. Their range in cm is about 50% of their energy in MeV, and their 80% isodose curve is about one-third of their energy in MeV. Thus a 6 MeV electron beam has its 80% isodose at 2 cm depth and a range of 3 cm. They are suitable for chest wall treatments, skin lesions and tumours which overlie critical organs.

Shielding blocks are used when a critical organ lies within or close to the treatment volume. These are often made of lead. Full shields are usually five or six half-value layers while partial transmission shields are one half-value layer.

2.4.6 Treatment planning methods

(a) Hand planning

Ideally, every treatment plan, except those with parallel plane fields, should be displayed with full isodose curves. However, this involves considerable work in departments with no planning computer. With experience, however, it is permissible to use appropriate fields known to give reasonable plans, without displaying the plan in full. Provided care is taken to check that only one field is going through a vital structure, e.g. spinal cord, this arrangement gives a satisfactory dose distribution and the dose can be prescribed at 2–3 cm depth with an equal contribution from each field.

(b) Computerized treatment planning

A dedicated planning computer is an essential item for every radiotherapy department, since manual computations are excessively time consuming and preclude the possibility of routinely comparing one field arrangement with another. A computer is not only better in speed of calculation, but also for teaching therapists in training and for developing consistent treatment policies by anatomical site.

A planning computer is just as important for radiotherapy departments in developing countries as for those in industrialized countries. For radical treatment, larger tumours are more complex to plan treatment for than early tumours, since the risk of damage to critical organs is greater.

The cancers with the highest incidence in developing countries include cancers of the nasopharynx, mouth, oesophagus, and cervix. All require accurate plans for optimal treatment. Planning computers are costly but various software packages are now available for use with personal computers which are much cheaper. Limitations of planning computers are that they do not reflect well the true field shaping resulting from lead blocks and also the isodoses in the build-up region.

2.4.7 Radiation therapy treatment sheet

For radiation therapy treatments to be accurate and reproducible, a treatment sheet must be used. This should contain the following minimum information.

Therapy machine
Machine identification, modality (electron or photon), beam energy (for orthovoltage, kV, added filtration and half-value layer).

Field details (for each field)
Name of site, diagram with any shielding or bolus indicated, patient thickness at central axis, depth of tumour, treatment distance (whether SSD or SAD), gantry, table and collimator orientation, wedge identification, immobilization device identification, calculation of treatment time or monitor setting for rotation therapy, the start and stop angles and dose per degree and preferably a photograph showing field marks and set-up.

Dose prescription
Technique (AP, PA, four-field brick, wedge pair, etc.), number of fields treated per day, daily tumour dose per field, total prescribed tumour dose, dose to critical structures, clear notes as to when the patient is to be re-evaluated, e.g. for field reduction, and the radiotherapist's name and signature.

Daily treatment record
Showing field identification, the day of treatment, time or monitor units set for each field daily and cumulative given (maximum) dose daily and cumulative tumour (target) dose from each field, daily and cumulative dose from all fields, critical structure dose, initials of person delivering the treatment.

Additional data
Isodose treatment plan and simulator verification films or port films which should be initialled by radiotherapist as satisfactory. Notes on any treatment interruptions, notes on previous irradiation, etc.

2.4.8 Immobilization devices

Immobilization devices are important for accurate reproducibility of the treatment position, especially in head and neck radiotherapy. A plaster impression is first made of the part to be treated and a perspex cast made from the plaster. The cast can then be screwed onto the treatment couch. Apart from immobilizing the patient, these devices have the advantage that field markings can be drawn on the cast rather than directly on the patient. This avoids unsightly marks on the body and also the marks on the cast are less likely to be washed off.

Since perspex is expensive, many centres in developing countries use simple devices, e.g. Sellotape, to check the patient's position but this is much less satisfactory since the angle of the head may vary from day to day. Other immobilization materials which are cheaper than perspex and may be reusable are being developed. The Orfit material (Thermoplast) is now becoming commercially available.

Young children present special problems. They may require sedation or even a general anaesthetic for the first few treatments, but this gradually improves with greater familiarity with the treatment room and staff.

2.4.9 Combined modality treatments

(a) Radiotherapy and chemotherapy

Many patients receive combined modality treatment. This is most commonly surgery and radiotherapy, but often radiotherapy and chemotherapy may be combined: radiotherapy for primary tumour control and chemotherapy for systemic micrometastasis (as in many paediatric cancers) or chemotherapy for primary control and radiotherapy for sanctuary sites (as in acute lymphatic leukaemia). All three modalities – surgery, radiotherapy and chemotherapy – are commonly used in paediatric cancers.

Care must be taken with combined modality treatments since toxicity may be potentiated. Chemotherapy may reduce renal, pulmonary or hepatic radiation tolerance and can increase skin reactions. Radiotherapy to the lumbar region may reduce bone marrow reserve and make subsequent chemotherapy more hazardous. Chemotherapy even months after radiotherapy can induce radiation side-effects (recall phenomenon), especially with actino-mycin D, adriamycin and bleomycin.

(b) External beam therapy and brachytherapy

Since brachytherapy involves giving a high dose to the primary tumour area, while external beam therapy enables a larger area to be treated to a less high dose, these two treatments may be usefully combined. For example, in the management of cancer of the cervix, external beam therapy to 45–50 Gy deals with the parametria and pelvic nodes involved, while intracavitary radiotherapy principally treats the primary tumour. Tongue tumours are often treated by preliminary external beam therapy to 40–50 Gy, with a further 30–40 Gy to the primary tumour area. Breast tumours may be treated in a similar way. Less commonly, many other sites can be treated with external beam–intracavitary treatment: bladder, naso-pharynx, lung, oesophagus, prostate, brain, etc.

Afterloading methods, whereby the radioactive source is loaded into the applicator after insertion into the patient, may be used at all the above sites, reducing radiation to staff. Remote-control after-loading methods are used especially with intracavitary treatments.

2.4.10 Large-field radiation

Large-field radiation may be used as total-body irradiation for bone marrow transplant patients, hemi-body irradiation for palliation of painful bone metastases, mantle irradiation in lymphomas, and irradiation of the whole central nervous system as in medulloblastoma.

These methods require large field sizes and thus an extended SSD, e.g. total-body irradiation for the treatment distance is over 3 m and with hemi-body irradiation it is about 1.5–2 m. Dose rates are low so treatment times are long. Full blood count should be checked previously. Anti-emetics, steroids and hydration may be required.

3

Head and neck

3.1 INCIDENCE AND RISK FACTORS

Head and neck cancer (HNC) comprises a diversity of tumour types and sites in the oral cavity, pharynx, larynx, paranasal sinuses, salivary glands and the thyroid. Of these, tumours arising in the mucosal epithelium are the most common. The incidence is highest in southern Asia and lowest in Japan with sharp variations in regions throughout the world, probably related to the variation in risk factors. The male to female ratio ranges from approximately 2 to 10.

Tobacco usage in its many forms (tobacco-betel quids, snuff, bidis (Indian mini-cigars), cigarettes, cigars and pipes) is the principal causative factor of oropharyngeal mucosal cancer. Associated, however, and a potent co-factor is alcohol, as well as poor oral hygiene. Nutritional deficiencies, particularly of vitamin A, are also probable co-factors.

Paranasal and nasopharyngeal cancers have been associated with wood dust and chemical fumes including various metals. Thyroid cancers have been associated with low-dose X-ray exposure and chronic iodine deficiencies.

3.2 PRESENTATION AND NATURAL HISTORY

The clinical presentation of early oral cancer is as a painless ulcer, proliferative growth, fissure with surrounding induration, velvety red patch or ulceration or induration in a pre-existing whitish patch anywhere in the oral cavity. When the lesion advances in the buccal mucosa it may produce skin ulceration, obliteration of the buccal sulci and expansion of the upper and lower alveoli. Trismus is a clinical manifestation of early lesions in the retromolar trigone and of many advanced malignant tumours in the head and neck. Superficial lesions on the dorsum of the tongue are white and papillomatous. Lateral margin lesions which are more posteriorly situated easily spread to the floor of the mouth and the base of the tongue. More infiltrative lesions restrict the mobility of the tongue.

Lower alveolar cancers present as localized painless ulcers or growths of the mucous membrane and may become painful with invasion of the bone and the periosteum.

Floor-of-mouth lesions are usually infiltrative and ulcerative and may produce extensive induration in the submaxillary and submandibular regions. Extension to the fraenulum of the tongue and lower alveolus is frequent in cancer of the floor of mouth.

Hard-palate lesions present as a thickening with surrounding reddish mucosa. Later they may extend to the maxillary antrum and may simulate cancer of the maxilla.

Distant metastasis is extremely uncommon in oral cancer. Lymphatic spread is most common in cancer of the tongue and the floor of the mouth and uncommon in early cancer of the buccal mucosa and palate. The lymph nodes involved are in the submandibular region and anterior cervical chain.

The predominant clinical symptom of oropharyngeal cancer is dysphagia. Small lesions in the base of the tongue and vallecula may be missed on clinical examination. Lesions in the faucial pillars extend easily to the palate, retromolar area and base of tongue. Lesions of the tonsil can extend to the lateral pharyngeal wall. Lymph node involvement is extremely frequent for this type of cancer (70%). The anterior cervical chain is predominantly involved even in comparatively early disease. Distant metastasis is not infrequent.

The predominant clinical feature of early cancer of the larynx is hoarseness of voice which is not relieved with conventional treatment. Stridor and dysphagia occur in later stages. In supraglottic cancer, these are delayed and pain referred to the ear may be the dominant symptom.

In early glottic cancer, lymphatic spread is rare, whereas lymphatic spread is common for supraglottic lesions and advanced glottic lesions.

The predominant initial symptom of hypopharyngeal cancer is dysphagia. Pyriform sinus lesions may not be detectable initially unless a direct examination is performed. Lymph node involvement is extremely common even in early states of the pyriform sinus cancer. Pain in the ear and hoarseness of voice are common in advanced disease. Advanced disease is invariably associated with massive lymph node disease and occasionally distant metastasis.

Nasopharyngeal neoplasms produce their clinical manifestations due to obliteration of the air cavity in the nasopharynx, and these include nasal twang, nasal obstruction and diminished hearing. Epistaxis due to ulceration, swelling in the oropharynx, displacement and ulceration of the soft palate, cranial nerve palsies, trismus and proptosis are prominent signs of this tumour. This tumour may occasionally have no obvious primary growth and the only manifestation may be enlargement of the anterior and posterior cervical lymph nodes. Distant metastasis to lung, bones and liver are common in nasopharyngeal cancer.

Patients with tumours in the middle ear have a long history of suppurative otitis media and the detection of malignant neoplasm is mostly accidental. Facial palsy is common.

Well-differentiated thyroid tumours present as a nodule in the thyroid, lymph node enlargement or a rapid increase in the size of a pre-existing thyroid nodule (goitre). Symptoms include dysphagia, hoarseness, voice stridor due to pressure, cough and bone pains due to lung and bone metastasis. The discovery of carcinoma may also be accidental when a cervical node is biopsied.

Well-differentiated papillary carcinomas of the thyroid occur predominantly in younger persons and are mostly asymptomatic. Lymphatic spread is the predominant pattern of spread. Haematogenous dissemination is rare. These are extremely slow-growing neoplasms.

Follicular thyroid cancer also presents as a nodule in the thyroid gland. These tumours metastasize with equal frequency in the central nervous system, lung and bone.

Anaplastic carcinomas are rapidly progressive tumours arising in a normal thyroid or a pre-existing goitre causing compressive and obstructive features leading to a medical emergency. They metastasize widely in the lymph nodes in neck and mediastinum, lung, liver and bones. They are extremely radiosensitive but do not take up radioiodine.

Medullary cancer of the thyroid also does not take up iodine but is moderately radiosensitive. Metastasis is predominantly to the lymph nodes in the neck and mediastinum. As this tumour arises from the perifollicular cells, it can be expected to produce a few paraneoplastic manifestations. However, these manifestations are not frequent. Thyroid lymphomas can be associated with gastrointestinal lymphoma.

The majority of swellings in the salivary glands are benign. The first evidence of malignant transformation is a rapid increase in size and facial palsy. Pain indicates rapid spread along the perineural pathways. Lymph node involvement is also rare and predominantly seen in muco-epidermoid cancer. Haematogenous spread to lungs is seen in adenoid cystic carcinoma. Such metastasis is not life-threatening and should not stand in the way of local therapy.

Malignant tumours constitute 25% of all parotid tumours. Malignant pleomorphic adenoma (pleomorphic adenocarcinoma) are the commonest malignant neoplasms in the parotid. Usually there will be a long history of a slow-growing parotid swelling which will start increasing in size rapidly and becoming painful.

Adenoid cystic carcinoma (cylindroma) is the commonest salivary malignant neoplasm (15%). These arise with equal frequency in the major, minor and ectopic salivary tissue especially the palate, upper alveolus, buccal mucosa, maxillary antrum and orbits. These tumours are slow-growing and spread along the perineural pathways which accounts for the unusual presentations of disease far away from the origin of the disease. Distant metastasis, especially pulmonary metastasis, is compatible with long life expectancy even without active therapy.

Squamous and anaplastic carcinoma of the salivary glands are either primary or metastasized from other skin or head and neck cancers. Primary squamous tumour of the salivary glands is highly malignant with an extremely poor prognosis whereas secondary tumours are amenable to therapy.

3.3 HISTOPATHOLOGY

Definite precancerous lesions can be identified in oral and laryngeal cancer. Three-quarters of invasive oral cancers originate in pre-existing leucoplakia which is a raised white path. Five to 15% of leucoplakias turn malignant within 15 years. Leucoplakias which are likely to turn malignant are the verrucous, erosive, speckled and nodular types, especially those situated in the lip, the floor of the mouth, and the lateral margins of the tongue. Another precancerous lesion is erythroplakia, which has a red velvet appearance. Submucous fibrosis is characterized by stiffening of the oral mucous membrane and consequent cracking and a parchment-like appearance.

Except in the thyroid and salivary glands, 95% of invasive cancers in the head and neck area are squamous carcinomas of varying differentiation.

Differentiated papillary, follicular cancers are the dominant histological types in the thyroid while anaplastic and medullary cancers constitute less than 10%.

Malignant mixed salivary tumours, adenoid cystic carcinoma and muco-epidermoid carcinoma are the dominant malignant tumours in major salivary glands and in the ectopic glands in the head and neck area.

3.4 INVESTIGATIONS

Mucosal lesions such as reddish patches, ulcers, proliferative growths, swelling, nodules, thickenings and indurated crevices should be viewed with suspicion. The minimal work-up in HNC includes a proper oral examination under good light, biopsy of the lesions, radiographs of the mandible/maxilla whenever indicated and complete blood counts. In the case of oro-, hypo- and nasopharyngeal and laryngeal cancers, endoscopic examination, biopsy and radiographs of the soft tissue of the neck are essential.

Nasopharyngoscopy, biopsy, X-rays of the base of skull and chest X-ray are mandatory in nasopharyngeal cancer. Excision biopsy, and X-rays of the chest are essential in salivary and thyroid cancers. Biopsy and X-rays of paranasal sinuses constitute the minimal work-up in maxillary sinus cancers. Liver function tests, renal function tests and complete blood counts are optional investigations in HNC. Histological confirmation of the lesions should be encouraged even in the presence of advanced cancers.

Thyroid nodules should be investigated with technetium 99M scans, if available, to determine their functional and pathological nature. Cold nodules should be investigated further with fine-needle aspiration or excision biopsy. In follicular cancer of the thyroid, whole-body profile scans will enable determination of metastatic sites.

Computed tomographic scan examination is helpful in maxillary cancer to decide the margins of surgical excision in operable cases and to plan radiotherapy in nasopharyngeal, nasal and middle ear tumours.

3.5 STAGING AND PROGNOSIS

The tumour, node, metastasis classification (TNM) is the most widely used system for recording the extent of local growth, regional and distant spread of HNC. The anatomical extent of disease is the prime indicator of prognosis for most cancer patients and provides the main criterion for selecting treatment.

The revised, unified 1987 formulation of the TNM classification published by the International Union Against Cancer and the American Joint Committee on Cancer is recommended for stage classification of HNC. The manual provides the details of anatomical subsites included in different sites, the regional lymph nodes, the rules for classification, TNM criteria, and stage grouping.

Table 3.1 provides the summary details of the TNM classification and stage groupings for HNC. The disease should be confirmed histologically before treatment. Physical examination and imaging are the procedures required for assessing the TNM categories.

Treatment results for various head and neck cancers indicate that the stage of the disease is one of the most important prognostic factors. The response rates and survival are invariably related to the clinical extent of disease in terms of composite stage, primary tumour size and the status of the regional lymph nodes (Table 3.2). Factors such as anatomical location of the tumour also influence survival. Location of the tumour has emerged as one of the independent prognostic factors in oral cancer. Lesions located in sites other than the buccal mucosa have a poorer prognosis, stage for stage. Similarly, lesions in supraglottis/subglottis demonstrate a poorer prognosis compared to glottic cancers. Post-cricoid cancers have a poorer prognosis compared with lesions in the pyriform fossa. Undifferentiated cancers of the thyroid fare poorly compared with differentiated cancers. Most salivary gland tumours have an indolent course.

Table 3.1 TNM classification for head and neck cancers (UICC, 1987)

	Primary tumours				Regional nodes		
	T1	T2	T3	T4	N1	N2	N3
Oral cavity	≤ 2 cm	2–4 cm	> 4 cm	Adjacent structure involvement	Ipsilateral single, ≤ 3 cm	Ipsilateral single, 3–6 cm	> 6 cm
Oropharynx	≤ 2 cm	2–4 cm	> 4 cm	Invades bone, muscle, etc.	Ipsilateral single, ≤ 3 cm	Ipsilateral multiple, ≤ 6 cm	> 6 cm
Nasopharynx	One subsite	More than one subsite	Invades nose/oropharynx	Invades skull/cranial nerve	Ipsilateral single, ≤ 3 cm	Bilateral, contralateral, ≤ 6 cm	> 6 cm
Ilypopharynx	One subsite	More than one subsite or adjacent site, without larynx fixation	With larynx fixation	Invades cartilage neck, etc.	Ipsilateral single, ≤ 3 cm	Bilateral, contralateral, ≤ 6 cm	> 6 cm
Glottis	One or both cords mobile	Extends to supra- or subglottis/ impaired	Cord fixation	Extends beyond larynx	Ipsilateral single, ≤ 3 cm	Bilateral, contralateral, ≤ 6 cm	> 6 cm
Supra- and subglottis	Limited to supraglottis/ subglottis, normal mobility	Extends in glottis, mobile	Cord fixation	Extends beyond larynx	Ipsilateral single, ≤ 3 cm	Bilateral, contralateral, ≤ 6 cm	> 6 cm
Salivary glands	≤ 2 cm	2–4 cm	4–6 cm	> 6 cm	Ipsilateral single, ≤ 3 cm	Bilateral, contralateral, ≤ 6 cm	> 6 cm
Maxillary sinus	Antral mucosa	Infrastructure, hard palate, nose	Cheek, floor of orbit, ethmoid, posterior wall of sinus	Orbital contents and other adjacent structures	Ipsilateral single, ≤ 3 cm	Bilateral, contralateral, ≤ 6 cm	> 6 cm
Thyroid gland	≤ 1 cm	1–4 cm	> 4 cm	Extends beyond gland	Regional node involvement	Not applicable	Not applicable

Table 3.2 Three-year survival rates (%) of patients with head and neck cancers by various stages in a regional cancer centre. Trivandrum (1982)

Stage	Buccal mucosa	Anterior tongue	Nasopharynx	Larynx
I	85	72	91	79
II	63	51	–	47
III	41	21	53	34
IV	15	19	30	15

3.6 TREATMENT – CHOICE OF MODALITY

3.6.1 Radical treatment

Small tumours of the head and neck are treatable adequately with either surgery or radiation and are equally curable with both modalities. As tumours in the head and neck region belong to the less radiosensitive group, only the small tumours which can be encompassed in small treatment volumes are curable with radiotherapy. Hence, early detection can improve the results of therapy. Radiotherapy is comparable to surgery in squamous cancer of the head and neck as it offers a reasonable chance for cure and palliation in all stages but avoids the disfiguring mutilation conferred by surgical resection. Non-squamous cell head and neck cancers with the exception of lymphomas are predominantly radioresistant, and surgery should invariably be used as the first line of management.

The success of radiotherapy in HNC will depend on the ability to give the maximum dose to the tumour without exceeding the tolerance of the normal tissues. If the volume treated is small, possibly less than 50 cm, it will be possible to give a very high dose with megavoltage radiation without damaging the normal tissues such as skin, soft tissues and bones. Moderately high doses with a good chance for cure can be administered if the area of the portal can be restricted to less than 100 cm. Volumes larger than these can be treated with radical doses only with a high probability of morbidity in the normal tissue.

The usual radical dose employed ranges from 50 Gy/15 fr/3 weeks to 66 Gy/33 fr/6$\frac{1}{2}$ weeks for most HNC.

Injury to the following normal tissues in the head and neck requires special mention when administering radical radiation. The susceptible tissues are the optic chiasma, brain stem, spinal cord, eyes and laryngeal cartilage, soft tissues of the oral cavity, mandible and conjunctiva.

3.6.2 Palliative treatment

Locally advanced HNC can benefit from palliative irradiation in order to control localized symptoms including respiratory compromise, functional difficulties in speech and swallowing, bleeding or discharge from exophytic tumours, cranial nerve involvement, and massive lymphadenopathy. Since most patients present with localized disease without evidence of distant metastases, aggressive radiation therapy using conventional, accelerated or hyperfractionated dose schedules is often administered. Dose fractionation schedules are also dependent on the radiation tolerance of the structures involved by tumour. The larynx is the most critical structure within the head and neck region since significant arytenoid oedema and airway compromise may result from doses exceeding 225 cGy per fraction or total doses of 60 Gy with conventional fractionation in cases without presenting tumour-related laryngeal inflammation. For this reason, hypofractionated irradiation is rarely applied in palliation of HNC. However, treatment of a tumour with extensive laryngeal involvement may require tracheostomy to maintain an adequate airway during radiation using any fractionation schedule.

The therapeutic approach in locally advanced HNC, including radiation fields and dose fractionation, generally follows principles used in definitive therapy. However, patients presenting with locally advanced disease and distant metastases may be treated with a more abbreviated dose fractionation schedule or systemic chemotherapy.

Tumours recurring within an area of previous external beam irradiation without distant disease are primarily approached with surgical salvage. Symptomatic recurrent disease associated with distant metastases which is unresponsive to systemic therapy may be palliated with either brachytherapy or further external beam irradiation combined with hyperthermia.

3.6.3 Other modalities

Surgery can be used either as the first line of management or for salvage. For small lesions in resectable sites, surgery is as effective as radiotherapy for cure, but can produce certain functional problems. Lesions whose volume is beyond radical radiotherapy are also best treated with surgery and followed up with post-operative radiotherapy for microscopic residual disease. In certain anatomical locations such as the tongue, surgical treatment gives better results. Such treatment is more expedient in older people. Salvage surgical excision is successful in 50% of all HNC patients and hence should be considered in radiotherapy failures when such a procedure will offer a reasonable quality of life. Operable lymph node disease is always better treated with surgical excision except when nodes are very small (< 3 cm). Such nodal masses can be sterilized with radiation in a significant proportion of cases.

3.7 RADIOTHERAPY TECHNIQUE

Whereas external beam from a 4 MV linear accelerator or telecobalt gamma rays are adequate for HNC in the majority of situations, some accessible lesions, especially those situated in the oral cavity, are treatable with brachytherapy or a combination of external beam therapy and brachytherapy.

Small lesions (T1, T2) in the commissural area of the buccal mucosa, lateral border of the tongue and even larger lesions of the lip are classic examples of lesions treatable with brachytherapy.

All small lesions (T1, T2) which are eccentrically situated in the head and neck area are treatable radically with the primary and lymph nodes in one volume with a wedge pair of fields or a combination of open and wedged fields. This has the advantage of limiting the radiation reaction to the target volume, thus reducing functional problems with swallowing, respiration, etc. The classic situations where this technique is applicable are the alveolus (upper and lower), the lateral margin of the tongue, the buccal mucosa, the maxillary antrum and the hard palate and tongue.

The same technique is suitable for small lesions (T1, T2) which lie anteriorly in the midline. Examples are floor-of-mouth and vocal cord lesions which are nearer to the anterior part of the contour.

Since the exit of beams can be adjusted to areas away from the vital structures, this technique permits delivery of high doses of radiation to the target volume.

In all moderately advanced lesions (T2, T3, T4) in situations where a large volume is to be irradiated by virtue of the need to treat the lymph nodes and when the disease is situated in the midline, a parallel opposing pair of fields is more convenient and quite adequate. The tumour doses achievable will be marginally lower with this technique because of tissue reactions. However, in the majority of the cases, radical treatment will be possible if a protracted fractionation is employed (25–30 fractions). Situations where such techniques are possible are cancers of the nasopharynx, tongue, hard palate, soft palate, oropharynx, larynx, and hypopharynx and radiotherapy for neck nodes.

Prophylactic neck radiation for micrometastasis can be carried out successfully with a single anterior open field.

Thyroid tumours which extend to the mediastinum are best treated with a parallel pair of angled (tipped) wedge fields to reach the lower limits of the disease.

3.7.1 Radical irradiation of neck nodes metastasis with unknown primary tumour

The target volume is all the cervical nodes. The prescribed dose is 50 Gy to this volume. The technique involves an anterior field with telecobalt and two posterior fields.

- *Position.* Supine with a neck rest in extension.
- *Field margins.* The field sizes are between 14×20 cm and 16×22 cm for the cervico supraclavicular field (Figure 3.1):

    upper limit: under the mastoid
    lower limit: 1 cm under the sternal notch
    lateral limits: internal middle of the clavicles

- *Beam modifications.* Median block to shield the larynx, and two blocks to shield the pulmonary apex.
- *Dose prescription.* The total dose at 2.5 cm is 44 Gy in 22 fractions over $4\frac{1}{2}$ weeks to the cervico supraclavicular field. The dose is increased to 50 Gy with three separated fields (one supraclavicular and two posterior cervical). The nodes with metastasis receive a boost of 10 Gy in 5 fractions with electrons if available.

3.7.2 Radical irradiation of supraclavicular nodes

The target volume is the inferior cervical nodes. The prescribed dose is 46 Gy to this volume. The technique involves an anterior field with telecobalt.

- *Position.* Supine with a neck rest in extension.
- *Field margins.* The field sizes are between 9×20 cm and 11×22 cm (Figures 3.2 and 3.3):

  upper limit: $\frac{1}{2}$ cm below the inferior limit of the lateral fields
  lower limit: 1 cm under the sternal notch
  lateral limits: internal middle of the clavicles

- *Beam modifications.* Median block to shield the larynx, and two blocks to shield the pulmonary apex.
- *Dose prescription.* The total dose at 3 cm is 46 Gy in 23 fractions over $4\frac{1}{2}$ weeks.

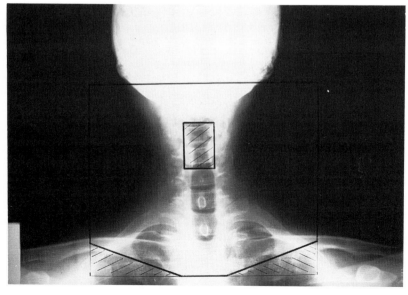

Figure 3.1 Radical irradiation of the cervical nodes. Outline of the field limits on a radiograph.

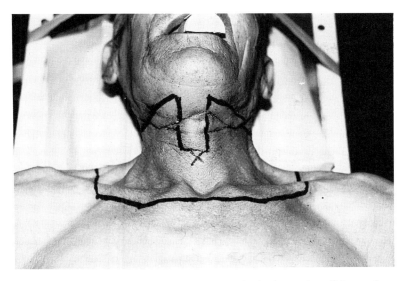

Figure 3.2 Radical irradiation of the supraclavicular nodes. Skin marks.

3.7.3 Radical irradiation for lateral tongue carcinoma with positive nodes

This is performed for T1 or T2 tumours 3 to 4 weeks after a neck nodes resection. The target volume is the tumour and the neck nodes. The prescribed dose is 68 Gy. The technique involves a pair of lateral opposed fields with telecobalt and an anterior field for the supraclavicular nodes.

- *Position*. Supine with a neck rest in semi-extension.
- *Field margins* (Figure 3.4).
  Large lateral fields:

  upper limit: hard palate
  lower limit: hyoid bone
  anterior limit: behind the mandible
  posterior limit: posterior profile of the neck

  Reduced lateral fields for tumour:

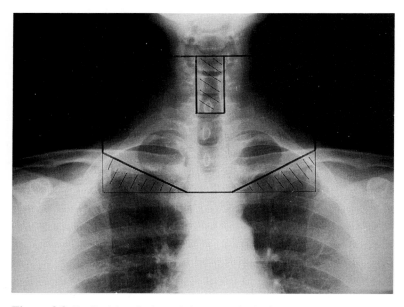

Figure 3.3 Radical irradiation of the supraclavicular nodes. Outline of the field limits on a radiograph.

> upper and lower limit: as above
> anterior limit: as above
> posterior limit: middle of the bodies of the vertebrae

Reduced lateral fields for spinal nodes with electrons of 9 MeV:

> upper and lower limit: as above
> anterior limit: middle of the bodies of the vertebrae
> posterior limit: posterior profile neck

- *Beam modifications.* Blocks to spare the brain.
- *Dose prescription* (Figures 3.5 and 3.6). The total dose at the axis intersection is 68 Gy in 34 fractions over $6\frac{1}{2}$ weeks on the tongue tumour with a reduction after 50 Gy to spare the oral cavity. After 40 Gy, a reduction to the spinal cord is performed. The dose is increased to 60 Gy if the nodes are invaded and to 50 Gy without invasion.
- *Special considerations* (Figure 3.7). If electrons are not available,

the dose to the spinal nodes can be performed with two posterior oblique fields with wedges. In this case, wedges are used on the reduced lateral fields for the tumour.

3.7.4 Radical irradiation of the oropharynx

This is performed for T1 or T2 tumours of the oropharynx. The target volume is the tumour and the cervical nodes. The prescribed dose is 64 Gy to the tumour and 50 Gy to the neck nodes without invasion. The technique involves a pair of lateral opposed fields with telecobalt and an anterior field for the supraclavicular nodes.

- *Position*. Supine with a neck rest in semi-extension.
- *Field margins* (Figure 3.8).
  Large lateral fields:

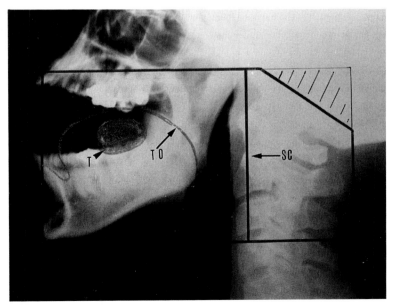

Figure 3.4 Radical irradiation of the lateral tongue. Outline of the field limits on a radiograph. T, tumour; TO, tongue; SC, spinal cord reduction.

upper limit: zygomatic arch
lower limit: hyoid bone
anterior limit: middle of the mandible
posterior limit: posterior profile of the neck

The reduced fields have the same limits as the lateral tongue carcinoma.

- *Beam modifications.* Blocks to spare the brain.
- *Dose prescription.* The total dose at the axis intersection is 64 Gy in 32 fractions over $6\frac{1}{2}$ weeks. A reduction for the spinal cord is performed after 40 Gy.
- *Special considerations.* If available, the dose can be limited to 50 Gy at the tumour and completed with brachytherapy (around 15 to 20 Gy).

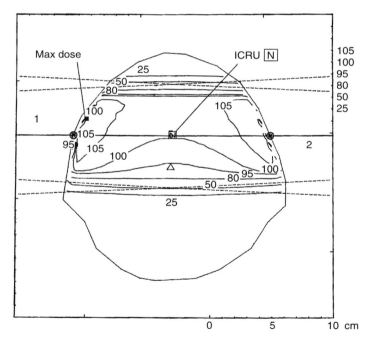

Figure 3.5 Radical irradiation of the lateral tongue after spinal cord reduction. Isodose distribution for cobalt and SSD = 80 cm. [N] normalized on the 100% (ICRU) point; (■) maximum dose 109%. Loading: (1) right lateral: 100 cGy/fr; (2) left lateral: 100 cGy/fr.

3.7.5 Radical irradiation for carcinoma of the buccal mucosa with negative nodes

The target volume is the lesion of the buccal mucosa and the homolateral inferior neck nodes. The prescribed dose is 64 Gy to the tumour volume and 46 Gy to the inferior neck nodes. The technique involves one anterior and one lateral orthogonal field with wedges for the buccal mucosa and a single hemi-anterior field for the neck nodes with telecobalt.

- *Position.* Lateral or supine with a neck rest in semi-extension.
- *Field margins* (Figures 3.9 and 3.10).
  Lateral fields (7 × 9 cm to 10 × 12 cm):

  upper limit: the superior part of the palate
  lower limit: horizontal ramus of the mandible

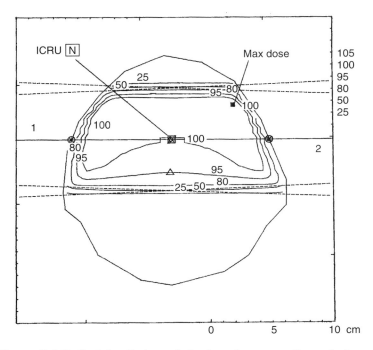

Figure 3.6 Radical irradiation of the lateral tongue after spinal cord reduction. Isodose distribution for 6 MV X-rays and SSD = 80 cm. [N] normalized on the 100% (ICRU) point; (■) maximum dose 104%. Loading: (1) right lateral: 100 cGy/fr; (2) left lateral, 100 cGy/fr.

anterior limit: commissure of the mouth
posterior limit: before the external meatus

Anterior field (7 × 7 cm to 10 × 9 cm):

upper and lower limit: as above
external limit: profile of the cheek
internal limit: midline of the mandible according to the extension of the lesion

- *Beam modifications.* Wedges of 45° must be positioned on the anterior and lateral fields.
- *Dose prescription* (Figure 3.11). The total dose at the axis intersection is 64 Gy in 32 fractions over 6½ weeks.
- *Special considerations.* If the nodes are invaded, the posterior limit of the lateral field is extended to the posterior profile neck. A reduction is performed for the spinal cord after 40 Gy.

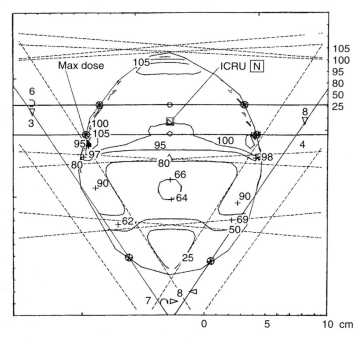

Figure 3.7 Radical irradiation of the lateral tongue and spinal nodes with two posterior oblique fields. Isodose distribution for cobalt and SSD = 80 cm. N normalized on the 100% (ICRU) point; (■) maximum dose 109%.

3.7.6 Radical irradiation of limited T1 glottic cancer

The target volume is the thyroid cartilage and the cricoid cartilage. The prescribed dose is 64 Gy to this volume. The technique involves a pair of lateral opposed fields with telecobalt.

- *Position.* Supine with a neck rest in semi-extension.
- *Field margins* (Figure 3.12). The field sizes are 5×5 cm to 6×6 cm:

      upper limit: under the hyoid bone
      lower limit: lower margin of cricoid cartilage
      anterior limit: profile of neck
      posterior limit: before the vertebral bodies

- *Beam modifications.* Wedges of 45° must be positioned on the fields.
- *Dose prescription* (Figure 3.13). The dose at the axis intersection is 64 Gy in 32 fractions over $6\frac{1}{2}$ weeks.

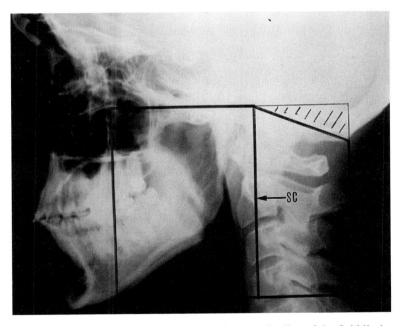

Figure 3.8 Radical irradiation of the oropharynx. Outline of the field limits on a radiograph. SC, spinal cord reduction.

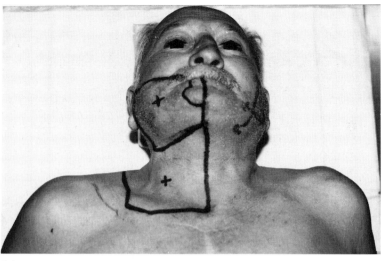

(a)

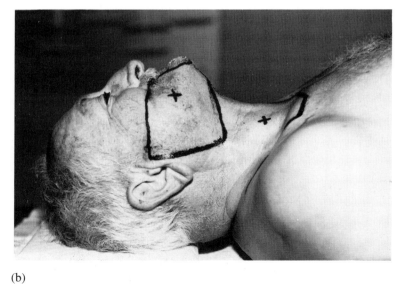

(b)

Figure 3.9 Radical irradiation of the buccal mucosa: skin marks. (a) Anterior field; (b) lateral field.

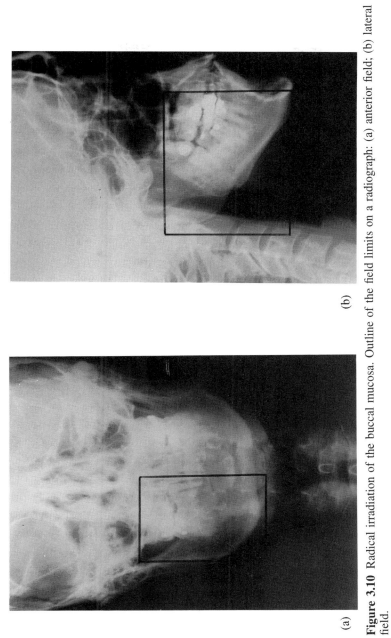

(a)

(b)

Figure 3.10 Radical irradiation of the buccal mucosa. Outline of the field limits on a radiograph: (a) anterior field; (b) lateral field.

- *Special considerations.* When the field sizes are more than 5 × 5 cm a reduction to exclude the arytenoid is performed after 60 Gy.

3.7.7 Radical irradiation for T1 supraglottic cancer

The target volume is the tumour and the neck nodes. The prescribed dose is 66 Gy to the tumour and 50 Gy to the neck nodes. The technique involves a pair of lateral opposed fields with telecobalt and an anterior field for the supraclavicular nodes.

- *Position.* Supine with a neck rest in semi-extension.
- *Field margins* (Figure 3.14). The field sizes are 13 × 10 cm to 15 × 11 cm:

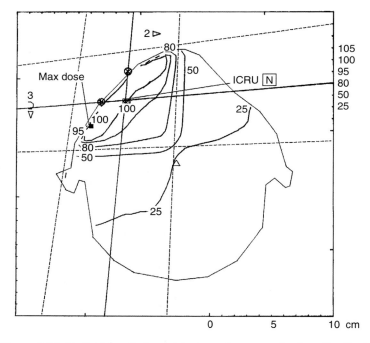

Figure 3.11 Radical irradiation of the buccal mucosa. Isodose distribution for cobalt and SSD = 80 cm. [N] normalized on the 100% (ICRU) point; (■) maximum dose 105%. Loading: (1, 2) anterior: 100 cGy/fr; (3, 4) lateral: 100 cGy/fr. One fraction with wedges and two fractions without wedges.

upper limit: above the angle of the mandible
lower limit: lower margin of cricoid cartilage
anterior limit: anterior profile of the neck
posterior limit: posterior profile of the neck

- *Beam modifications.* Block on the angle of the mandible to spare the oropharynx.
- *Dose prescription.* The total dose at the axis intersection is 66 Gy in 33 fractions over $6\frac{1}{2}$ weeks. After 40 Gy a reduction to the spinal cord is performed.

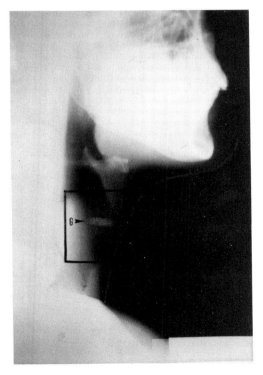

Figure 3.12 Radical irradiation of limited glottic cancer. Outline of the field limits on radiograph. G, glottic airspace.

3.7.8 Radical irradiation alone for carcinoma of the nasopharynx

The target volumes are the nasopharynx and the upper and lower neck nodes. The prescribed dose is 60 Gy to the tumour and 50 Gy to the lymph nodes. The technique involves a pair of lateral opposed fields for the nasopharynx with a reduction after 50 Gy and a single anterior field for the neck with telecobalt.

- *Position.* Supine with an appropriate neck rest in semi-extension.
- *Localization.* Marks on lateral margin of the orbit and over a node mass
- *Field margins* (Figure 3.15).
  Nasopharynx lateral fields:

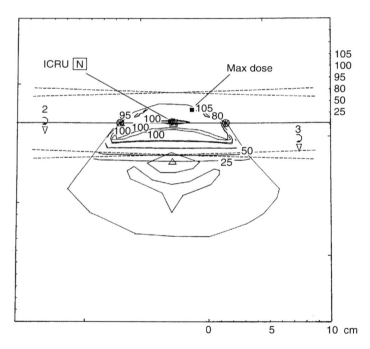

Figure 3.13 Radical irradiation of limited glottic cancer. Isodose distribution for cobalt and SSD = 80 cm. $\boxed{\text{N}}$ normalized on the 100% (ICRU) point; (■) maximum dose 105%. Loading: (1, 2) right lateral: 100 cGy/fr; (3, 4) left lateral: 100 cGy/fr. One fraction with wedges and two fractions without wedges.

upper limit: superior orbital margin
lower limit: hyoid bone
anterior limit: lateral orbital margin
posterior limit: profile of the neck

Nasopharynx reduced lateral fields:

upper and anterior limit: as above
lower limit: occlusal plane of the mouth
posterior limit: line of external auditory meatus

Nodes anterior field:

upper limit: hyoid bone
lower limit: sternal notch
lateral limit: profile of the neck

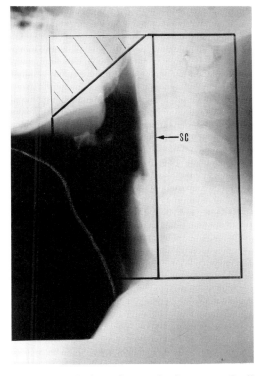

Figure 3.14 Radical irradiation of supraglottic cancer. Outline of the field limits on radiograph.

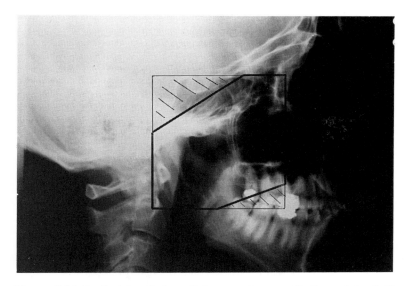

Figure 3.15 Radical irradiation of the nasopharynx. Outline of the field limits on radiograph.

- *Beam modifications.* Blocks on lateral fields to spare the brain and the oral cavity, and blocks on the anterior field to spare the larynx and pulmonary apex.
- *Dose prescription.* For the nasopharynx, the total dose at the axis intersection is 60 Gy in 30 fractions over 6 weeks with a reduction after 50 Gy. For the neck nodes, the dose at 3 cm is 46 Gy in 23 fractions over $4\frac{1}{2}$ weeks.

3.7.9 Radical irradiation for ethmoid carcinoma with negative nodes

This is performed for T1, T2 or T3 tumours 3 to 4 weeks after a neck nodes resection. The target volume is the tumour and the neck nodes. The prescribed dose is 64 Gy to the tumour volume and 50 Gy to the neck nodes. The technique involves one anterior and two lateral orthogonal fields with wedges for the tumour and the nodes and one reduced anterior field for the tumour with telecobalt.

- *Position.* Supine with a neck rest in semi-extension with head contention if available.
- *Field margins* (Figures 3.16 and 3.17).
  Anterior field (7–8 cm × 4–5 cm):

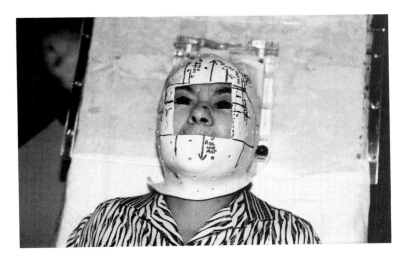

(a)

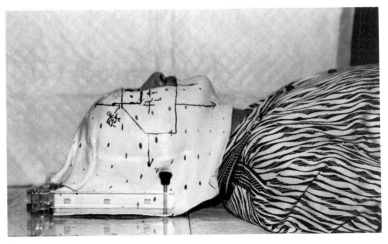

(b)

Figure 3.16 Radical irradiation of the ethmoid. Skin marks: (a) anterior field; (b) lateral field.

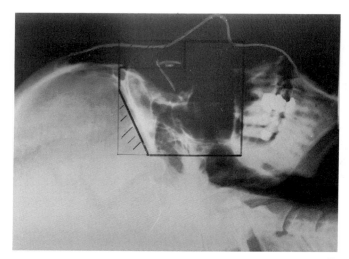

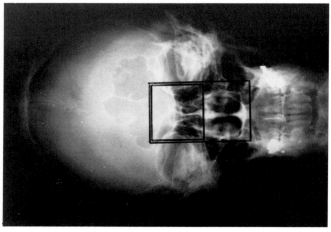

(b)

(a)

Figure 3.17 Radical irradiation of the ethmoid. Outline of the field limits on a radiograph: (a) anterior field; (b) lateral field.

upper limit: superior orbital margin
lower limit: superior part of the palate
external limit: internal orbital margin

Lateral fields (7–8 cm × 8–9 cm):

upper and lower limits: as above
anterior limit: anterior of nasal cavity
posterior limit: anterior of anterior clinoid

Anterior reduced field (4–5 cm × 4–5 cm):

upper and external limit: as above
lower limit: inferior orbital margin

- *Beam modifications.* Blocks to spare the brain and the eyes on the lateral fields.
- *Dose prescription* (Figure 3.18). The total dose at the axis

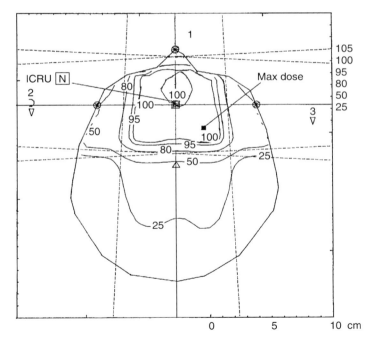

Figure 3.18 Radical irradiation of the ethmoid. Isodose distribution for cobalt and SSD = 80 cm. $\boxed{N}$ normalized on the 100% (ICRU) point; (■) maximum dose 105%.

intersection is 50 Gy in 25 fractions over 5 weeks for the neck nodes. The tumour is boosted with 14 Gy in 7 fractions over $1\frac{1}{2}$ weeks on a reduced field.

3.7.10 Radical post-operative irradiation for thyroid

This is performed 4–6 weeks after radical surgery in cases of high risk of recurrence in the tumour bed (thyroid area) or in the neck nodes area. The target volume is the thyroid area, upper retrosternal and supraclavicular nodes, and the bilateral neck nodes. The pre-scribed dose is 60 Gy (56–60 Gy) in the thyroid area and 50 Gy in the nodal areas. Great care is taken not to give a dose of more than 40 Gy (44 Gy) to the spinal cord. The technique is a difficult one with cobalt alone involving a large anterior field with two posterior oblique fields to increase the dose to the lateral and posterior part of the neck nodes.

- *Position.* Supine with a neck rest in extension.
- *Localization.* Lead marker to delineate the upper part of the larynx.
- *Field margins* (Figure 3.19).
  Large anterior field (complex shape, approximately 18 cm high and 23 cm wide):

  upper limit: under the mastoid and mandible
  lower limit: 5 cm below the sternal notch
  lateral limits: middle of clavicles

  Posterior oblique field (13 × 7 cm) treated through the table (or patient in prone position):

  upper limit: mastoid
  lower limit: clavicle
  outer limit: skin margins
  inner limit: lead marker on the anterior part of the neck 1 cm lateral to the midline

- *Beam modifications.* The anterior field is treated with an SSD of 80 cm. A lead block is positioned at the upper part of the larynx to shield the upper part of the larynx and the submental area. The posterior fields are tilted 5° inferiorly. They are treated with a SAD technique. The isocentre of the cobalt is 2.5 cm below the mid-jugular nodes. The gantry is 175° or 185° if the patient is prone. A 45° wedge is positioned in the posterior field.

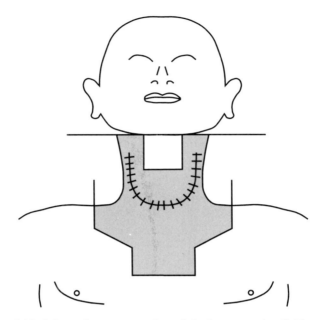

Figure 3.19 Schematic representation of the large anterior field.

- *Dose prescription* (Figures 3.20 and 3.21). The dose to the anterior field is 200 cGy per fraction (usually 5 mm below the surface of the skin). The total dose is 56 Gy in 28 fractions over 6 weeks (given dose). The posterior fields are treated only twice. A dose of 200 cGy per fraction is given at the mid-jugular node. The total dose is 4 Gy in 2 fractions. With such a technique, the spinal cord does not receive more than 40 Gy with standard anatomy.
- *Special consideration.* If there is no surgery the dose to the anterior field may be increased to 60 Gy and the dose to the posterior fields to 8 Gy. The dose to the spinal cord must be kept below 45 Gy.

3.8 MORBIDITY

Inflammation of mucosal surfaces (mucositis) occurs routinely during head and neck irradiation. Symptoms include xerostomia, pain in the throat and on swallowing which can further compromise

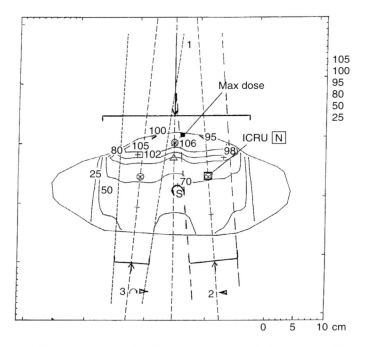

Figure 3.20 Post-operative irradiation, anterior field. Isodose distribution through the thyroid area (lower slice) for cobalt and SSD = 80 cm. $\boxed{\text{N}}$ normalized in the central axis slice on the mid-jugular node (2.5 cm below the skin); (■) maximum dose 117%. The 100% isodose receives 50 Gy. The maximum dose is 58 Gy. The dose to the spinal cord is less than 40 Gy. Fields (2) and (3) are the two oblique posterior fields with 45° wedges.

nutritional intake. Local effects of the tumour reported in < 25% of patients with HNC, including pain and difficulties in swallowing, are exacerbated temporarily during irradiation. The aetiology of the mucositis is multifactorial including radiation injury and infection. During the course of therapy, changes in the flora within the oropharynx include a larger percentage of Gram-negative organisms and *Candida* species. Antimicrobial agents including chlorhexidine, benzydamine, and nystatin have been administered in attempts to reduce the degree of inflammation, but no consistent impact of analgesia has been reported. Using topical anaesthetics and codeine elixirs, pain associated with mucositis can be reduced. Improved

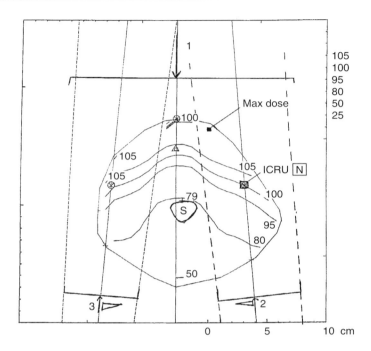

Figure 3.21 Post-operative irradiation, anterior field. Isodose distribution through the mid-jugular node (central axis slice) for cobalt and SSD = 80 cm. [N] normalized in the central axis slice on the mid-jugular node (2.5 cm below the skin); (■) maximum dose 116%. The 100% isodose receives 50 Gy. The dose to the spinal cord is less than 40 Gy (S).

management of mucosal symptoms has been reported with daily clinical assessments and aggressive treatments of pain utilizing a three-step analgesic protocol based on the severity of symptoms, resulting in effective pain relief in 94% of patients and a reduction in weight loss under treatment. Aggressive nutritional support including dietary supplementation either with oral intake or naso-gastric feeding is critical to maintain hydration and allow repair of normal tissues. Optimization of oral hygiene acts to reduce oral flora, thickened secretions and debris, and increase moisture within the mouth.

4

Oesophagus

4.1 INCIDENCE AND RISK FACTORS

Approximately 50% of oesophageal carcinomas arise in the middle third of the oesophagus, and 25% arise in the upper and lower thirds respectively. The incidence and mortality of oesophageal carcinoma vary in different parts of the world, being lowest in Canada (2.2/100 000) and highest in northern China (109/100 000). Other high incidence areas are South Africa, Iran, and the western part of France. According to a nationwide survey of cancer mortality, oesophageal cancer ranks second in men and third in women among the common cancers in China. The mortality from oesophageal cancer is higher in rural areas than in cities. Alcoholism associated with cigarette smoking and disorders in dietary habits (diet low in animal protein and fat, with lower consumption of vegetables and fruits) are the main aetiological factors.

4.2 PRESENTATION AND NATURAL HISTORY

Dysphagia is the leading symptom in all patients but unfortunately, it is a late one. The chief complaints during early oesophageal cancer are a sense of stenosis and chest pain on swallowing. At the median or late stage of oesophageal cancer, the symptoms are dysphagia in 98%, weight loss in 51%, retrosternal pain in 33%, regurgitation/vomiting in 23%, cough in 7% and hoarseness in 3%.

The gross pattern of oesophageal cancer may be divided into fungating, infiltrating and ulcerative types. Fungating carcinoma is found in about 55% of cases. Its main feature is a prominent intraluminal growth, forming a mass with some ulceration or multiple polypoid excrescences. Infiltrating carcinoma is seen in about 25% of cases and shows primarily as intramural growth of the tumour which is always extensive under the intact mucosa at its periphery. Ulcerative carcinoma constitutes about 20% of cases. The ulcer has a variable depth. It always penetrates through the wall into the mediastinum or the peripheral organs, firstly the trachea and bronchus.

Metastases to lymph nodes are present in about 50% of cases. Metastases to distant organs were found only in those cases with lymph node involvement. The liver and lung are the organs most often involved.

4.3 HISTOPATHOLOGY

Squamous cell carcinoma is the most common tumour in the oesophagus (> 90%). The much less common adenocarcinoma usually occurs at the lower end of the oesophagus in close association with gastric epithelium.

4.4 INVESTIGATIONS

The necessary investigations include:

- a barium meal of upper gastrointestinal tract;
- endoscopy with biopsy;
- a computed tomographic scan of the mediastinum and abdomen to evaluate lymph node involvement, the peri-oesophageal situation, and hepatic metastases;
- post-operative pathological investigation including the size (length) of the tumour and its extent into peripheral structures, whether the margins of surgical specimen are tumour-free, and the status of lymph nodes (number, site); and
- careful examination of the lymph nodes of the neck, especially the supraclavicular, before operation and radiotherapy.

4.5 STAGING AND PROGNOSIS

The clinical TNM–UICC classification is identical to the pathological (post-surgical) classification but it is not always easy to assess the status of the mediastinal lymph nodes and the situation of peri-oesophageal structures accurately (Table 4.1).

Table 4.1 Classification of oesophageal carcinoma (UICC, 1987)

Stage	Description
TX	Primary tumour cannot be assessed
T0	No evidence of primary tumour
Tis	Carcinoma *in situ*
T1	Tumour invades lamina propria or submucosa
T2	Tumour invades muscularis propria
T3	Tumour invades adventitia
T4	Tumour invades adjacent structures
NX	Regional lymph nodes cannot be assessed
N0	No regional lymph node metastasis
N1	Regional lymph node metastasis
MX	Presence of distant metastasis cannot be assessed
M0	No distant metastasis
M1	Distant metastasis

Table 4.2 Results of treatment of oesophageal carcinoma

	Radical surgery alone	Radical radiotherapy alone	No treatment
Median survival	16 months	9–12 months	4–6 months
Five-year survival	N0, 40–60% N1, < 10%	< 10%	25%

Prognosis is very poor mainly because of contiguous extension of the carcinoma beyond the oesophageal wall and the close relationships with surrounding structures. It is thus difficult to radically resect the tumour. In recent years, radiotherapy has significantly changed the treatment policy towards this tumour and has provided some symptomatic relief, but has not improved the pessimistic outcome. Table 4.2 gives the predicted survival time according to treatment and stages.

4.6 TREATMENT – CHOICE OF MODALITY

4.6.1 Radical treatment

Surgery is the essential treatment of choice for early cases of oesophageal cancer (T1–T2 N0). The only hope of a cure for carcinoma of the oesophagus is resection of the tumour. However, less than 50% of the patients are appropriate candidates for surgery, as the tumour is widespread locally at the time of detection in the majority of patients.

As far as we know, there is no evidence of any benefit from postoperative irradiation in improving the long-term survival rate for oesophageal cancer. When the patient is curable but inoperable, radiotherapy is the essential treatment of choice, eventually combined with chemotherapy. Combination approaches with *cis*-platinum are promising.

4.6.2 Palliative treatment

In T3 and T4 cancers or regardless of the primary tumour staging if any lymphatic or distant metastases have occurred, radical treatment is useless. Bypass operations can be performed for severe dysphagia. Endoscopic laser, intraluminal intubation and endoluminal brachytherapy are additional palliative methods.

In the case of oesophageal obstruction with a poor nutritional situation due to long-term starvation and dehydration, these conditions must be corrected with total parenteral nutrition and/or gastrostomy in order to complete the full course of planned palliative radiotherapy.

4.7 RADIOTHERAPY TECHNIQUES

4.7.1 Radical irradiation alone

This is performed in patients with T1 or T2 tumours with no metastatic involvement who have a medical contra-indication for surgery. The target volume includes the tumour, with a safety margin of 4 cm on each extremity, and peritumoral mediastinal nodes. The prescribed dose is 54 Gy to the mediastinum and 64 Gy to the oesophagus. The method is a four-field box technique with telecobalt.

- *Position*. Supine.
- *Localization*. Barium in the oesophagus.
- *Field margins* (Figures 4.1 and 4.2).

Anterior and posterior fields (15 × 7 cm to 20 × 9 cm):

upper and lower limits: 4 cm around the tumour
lateral limits: 2 cm around the oesophagus

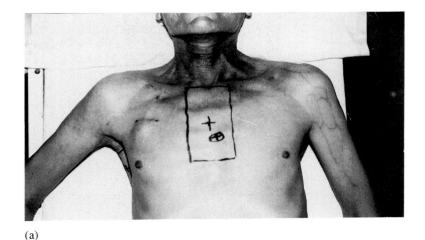

(a)

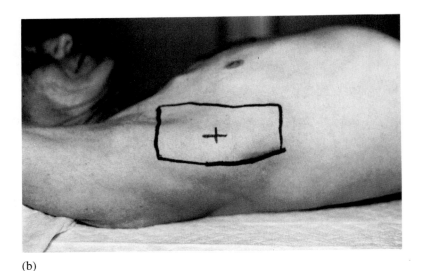

(b)

Figure 4.1 Radical irradiation. Skin marks: (a) anterior field; (b) lateral field.

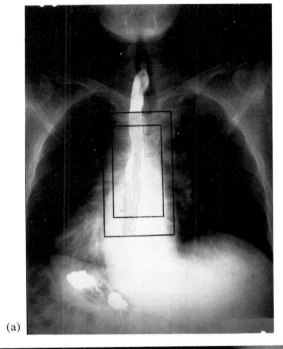

(a)

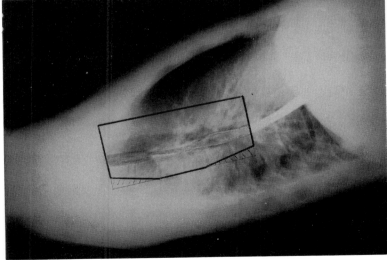

(b)

Figure 4.2 Radical irradiation. Outline of the field limits on a radiograph: (a) anterior field and reduced field; (b) lateral field.

Lateral fields (15 × 6 cm to 20 × 8 cm):

upper and lower limits: 4 cm around the tumour
lateral limits: 2 cm around the oesophagus
anterior limit: 2 cm anterior to the oesophagus
posterior limit: 1 cm behind the anterior wall of the vertebral
body

- *Beam modifications.* Blocks on the lateral fields to protect the spinal cord if irradiated.
- *Dose prescription* (Figures 4.3 and 4.4). The dose on the mediastinum is 54 Gy in 27 fractions over $5\frac{1}{2}$ weeks. After 3 weeks rest, a boost of 10 Gy in 5 fractions over 1 week is given with rotation therapy on a reduced field.
- *Special consideration.* An alternative is a three-field arrangement (one anterior and two oblique posterior).

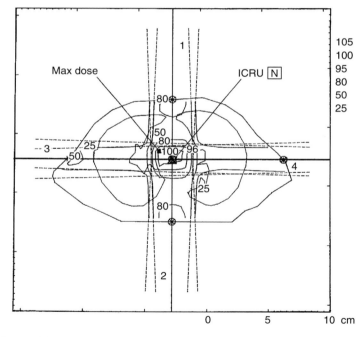

Figure 4.3 Radical irradiation. Isodose distribution for cobalt and SSD = 80 cm. ⟦N⟧ normalized on the 100% (ICRU) point; (■) maximum dose 103%. Loading: (1) anterior: 80 cGy/fr; (2) posterior: 80 cGy/fr; (3) right lateral: 20 cGy/fr; (4) left lateral: 20 cGy/fr.

4.7.2 Palliative radiotherapy

This is used to palliate symptoms such as dysphagia. The target volume is the tumour of the oesophagus. A simple technique with AP–PA fields and moderate dose is recommended.

- *Position.* Supine.
- *Localization.* Barium in the oesophagus.
- *Field margins.*
  Anterior and posterior fields (15×7 cm to 20×9 cm):

  upper and lower limits: 4 cm around the tumour
  lateral limits: 2 cm around the oesophagus

- *Dose prescription* (Figure 4.5). 30 Gy in 10 fractions, 5 fractions per week.

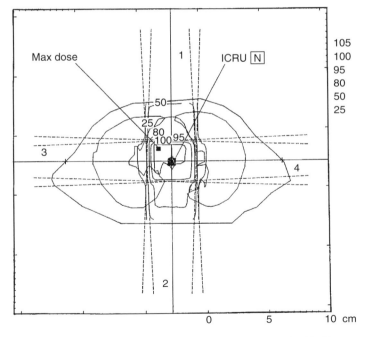

Figure 4.4 Radical irradiation. Isodose distribution for 18 MV X-rays and SAD = 100 cm. N normalized on the 100% (ICRU) point; (■) maximum dose 100%. Loading: (1) anterior: 80 cGy/fr; (2) posterior: 80 cGy/fr; (3) right lateral: 20 cGy/fr; (4) left lateral: 20 cGy/fr.

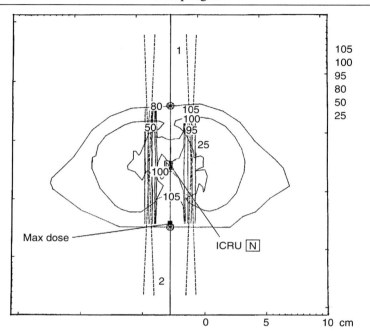

Figure 4.5 Radical irradiation. Isodose distribution for cobalt and SSD = 80 cm. N normalized on the 100% (ICRU) point; (■) maximum dose 118%. Loading: (1) anterior: 150 cGy/fr; (2) posterior: 150 cGy/fr.

4.8 MORBIDITY

Most patients develop radiation oesophagitis approximately three weeks after the start of radiotherapy. Continued retrosternal pain, fever and persistent haematemesis all suggest oesophageal perforation. If an oesophagogram confirms the perforation, irradiation should be discontinued.

Overdosage irradiation may lead to oesophageal stenosis and produces symptoms that mimic the original tumour. Perforation and haemorrhage are usually due to tumour destruction by irradiation. Late stenosis is not unusual in patients whose tumours have been controlled by irradiation.

5

Lung

5.1 INCIDENCE AND RISK FACTORS

Lung cancer is a worldwide problem, with a steady increase in both sexes but its incidence is highest in industrial countries. Scotland, England, Wales and Finland have the highest incidences of lung cancer, while the United States ranks 10th and Mexico ranks 37th among the 40 countries surveyed. Some studies have shown that the rate of increase of incidence of lung cancer is higher in women than in men.

The main aetiological factor is inhaled tobacco smoke. Other carcinogenic substances (e.g. abestos) that cause lung cancer are also being identified, especially in the work place.

5.2 PRESENTATION AND NATURAL HISTORY

Signs and symptoms in lung cancer patients depend on the site and size of the primary tumour and on the metastatic potential of the neoplasm for regional location (hilar and mediastinal nodes) or for distant metastasis. While the majority of bronchogenic carcinomas arise in peripheral bronchi, epidermoid carcinoma and small-cell anaplastic carcinomas have generally extended centrally by the time of clinical presentation. In these cell types endoscopy often reveals fungating lesions in mainstem, lobar or proximal segmental bronchi. In contrast, adenocarcinoma generally remains peripheral and is identified less often on endoscopy. Large-cell anaplastic carcinoma is also often located peripherally, but it tends to form larger tumour masses than does adenocarcinoma.

Symptoms secondary to central and endobronchial tumour growth are cough, dyspnoea, chest pain, haemoptysis, wheeze or stridor, and pneumonia (fever, productive cough). Symptoms caused by regional lesions are nerve involvement, including the recurrent laryngeal nerve (hoarseness) and phrenic nerve (hemidiaphragmatic elevation with dyspnoea). Vascular compression due to lung cancer may cause superior vena cava syndrome, pericardial or cardiac extension arrhythmia or cardiac failure. Mediastinal extension of the cancer may cause dysphagia (oesophageal compression) and pleural effusion (lymphatic obstruction). Apical pulmonary carcinoma may lead to severe pain of the arm and shoulder, due to Pancoast syndrome.

The natural history of lung cancer encompasses three stages:

1. a period of months to years during which increasing degrees of cellular atypia are noted on sputum cytological examination,
2. a period of variable duration characterized by progression of cytologic atypia to carcinoma *in situ*, and
3. a period of clinically evident tumour. Only during this latter phase does one note signs and symptoms related to local, regional or systemic dissemination of the tumour or to development of systemic paraneoplastic symptoms unrelated to tumour sites.

Depending on the TNM staging, histopathology, the patient's general condition, and the biological behaviour of the tumour at the time of diagnosis, an untreated patient will have an average survival time of 3–6 months. The cause of death is due to the effects of primary tumour on airway and vasculature or the progression of distant metastases in vital organs or both.

5.3 HISTOPATHOLOGY

The four major cell types include epidermoid carcimona, adenocarcinoma, small-cell and large-cell carcinoma. If strict criteria are applied for diagnosis, about 2–4% of these tumours will be found to be composed of a combination of glandular and squamous epithelium.

5.4 INVESTIGATIONS

The basic laboratory investigation in addition to the complete history and physical examination is the posterior–anterior lateral

Table 5.1 TNM classification of lung carcinoma (UICC, 1987)

Stage	Description
TX	Positive cytology
T1	$\leqslant 3$ cm
T2	> 3 cm/extends to hilar region/invades visceral pleura/ partial atelectasis
T3	Chest wall, diaphragm, pericardium, mediastinal pleura, etc., total atelectasis
T4	Mediastinum, heart, great vessels, trachea, oesophagus, etc., malignant effusion
N1	Peribronchial, ipsilateral hilar nodes
N2	Ipsilateral mediastinal nodes
N3	Contralateral mediastinal, scalene or supraclavicular nodes

chest radiograph, on which the preliminary diagnosis is usually made. When available, a chest computed tomographic examination is performed, which should also include the upper abdomen (liver and adrenal glands). The tissue diagnosis is made by one or more of the following increasingly invasive procedures:

- sputum cytology – spontaneous or induced sputum production
- bronchoscopy
- mediastinoscopy
- fluoroscopically guided fine-needle aspiration
- transthoracic wall biopsy
- thoracotomy

Staging of a patient with small-cell anaplastic carcinoma may include additionally radionuclide bone scanning and brain computed tomography.

5.5 STAGING AND PROGNOSIS

Table 5.1 shows the TNM system for lung cancer staging. Surgery and curative radiotherapy are applicable to local or regional tumours only. T1N0M0 patients have a somewhat better prognosis than those with T2N0M0 tumours. Either will have a better prognosis than patients with small tumours and positive regional nodes (T1N1M0). The results of resection in stage III epidermoid and large-cell carcinomas with positive mediastinal nodes are hardly outstanding, but they are superior to the results achieved by other primary treatment modalities.

As far as we know, there has been no significant improvement of five-year survival after use of telecobalt or other supervoltage irradiation. However, gratifying palliation, often dramatic, can be achieved in about 75% of patients.

In recent years, combined therapeutic approaches, the use of radiosensitizers, and change of routine time–dose relationship have developed, but need to be fully explored. The five-year survival is still less than 10%.

5.6 TREATMENT – CHOICE OF MODALITY

5.6.1 Radical treatment

Since there is no single uniformly effective treatment against lung cancer, there must be a spirit of cooperation among surgical, medical and radiation oncologists. In this tumour the job of the radiotherapist is to cure some patients and to palliate many.

5.6.2 Palliative treatment

Palliation remains a significant aspect of lung cancer management, despite the therapeutic approach, since the majority of patients are symptomatic at presentation due to the lack of reliable screening techniques. The role of palliative irradiation of lung cancer is broad. Clinical presentations associated with carcinoma of the lung include dyspnoea, cough, haemoptysis, post-obstructive pneumonia, pain and superior vena cava obstruction. Included is the definitive treatment of a symptomatic locally advanced lesion without associated distant metastases using conventional or other aggressive fractionation schedules. This approach is based on the significant decrease in histologically evident tumour destruction at autopsy reported after hypofractionated irradiation. A similar aggressive treatment approach is advocated for primary clinical presentations with superior vena cava syndrome since 15% of patients survive for longer than two years. An initial dose of 400 cGy is often administered in patients with significant manifestations of the syndrome followed by conventional fractionation to a total dose of 60–70 Gy. Radiotherapeutic management of malignant pleural effusion requires hemithoracic irradiation. As irradiation is limited by tolerance of the uninvolved areas of the lung to a total dose of 20 Gy with conventional fractionation, techniques including electron beam therapy have been utilized; however, dosimetry with this approach is complicated and overall prognosis poor. Symptom management with evacuation of the pleural fluid and use of sclerosing agents is generally applied.

Recurrent carcinoma in a previously irradiated volume or untreated primary disease associated with distant metastases at presentation is usually approached with hypofractionated irradiation (usually totalling 30 Gy in 10 fractions), although conventional fractionation totalling 40–50 Gy has been applied to small volumes resulting in 48% of patients reporting improvement of symptoms and a 74% objective response rate. Interstitial irradiation has been used with greater frequency to palliate obstructive symptoms in locally recurrent endobronchial lesions.

5.7 RADIOTHERAPY TECHNIQUES

5.7.1 Radical radiotherapy alone

This is performed in cases of T1 or T2 non-small-cell carcinoma of the lung without nodal involvement. The target volume is the tumour, the mediastinum and the supraclavicular nodes. The prescribed dose is 74 Gy to the tumour. The technique is a four-field box technique with telecobalt.

- *Position.* Supine with the arms raised on the head.
- *Supraclavicular field margins.* As for head and neck cancer.
- *Lung and mediastinum field margins* (Figures 5.1 and 5.2).
  Anterior and posterior fields:

  upper limit: joint with the supraclavicular field
  lower limit: about 4 cm below the carina
  lateral limits: 1 cm of the vertebral bodies on the opposite side of the tumour, 2–3 cm of the tumour on the side of the tumour

  Lateral fields:

  upper and lower limits: as above
  anterior and posterior limits: a safety margin of about 2–3 cm around the tumour

- *Beam modifications.* Blocks on AP–PA fields.

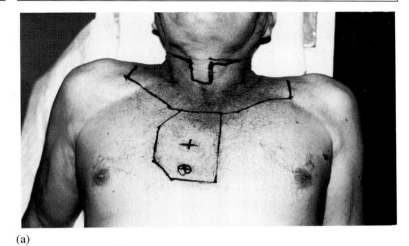

(a)

(b)

Figure 5.1 Radical irradiation. Skin marks: (a) anterior field and supraclavicular field; (b) lateral field.

- *Dose prescription* (Figure 5.3). The total dose at the axis intersection is 54 Gy in 27 fractions over $5\frac{1}{2}$ weeks.
- *Special considerations* (Figure 5.4). After a rest of 3 weeks,
10 Gy are added on a reduced boost field with a rotation therapy
technique. The dose to the spinal cord is limited to 40–45 Gy.

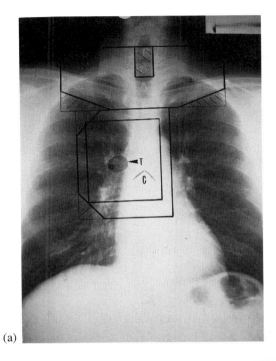

(a)

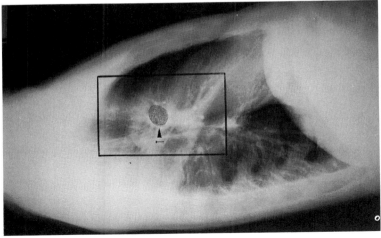

(b)

Figure 5.2 Radical irradiation. Outline of the field limits on a radiograph: (a) anterior, reduced and supraclavicular fields; (b) lateral field. T, tumour; C, carina.

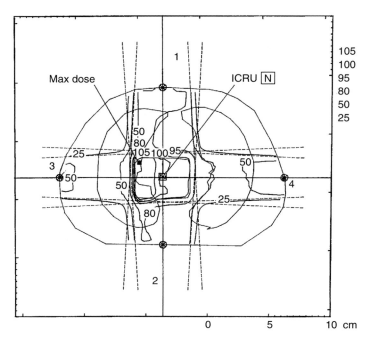

Figure 5.3 Radical irradiation. Isodose distribution for cobalt and SSD = 80 cm. ▢N▢ normalized on the 100% (ICRU) point; (■) maximum dose 119%. Loading: (1) anterior: 70 cGy/fr; (2) posterior: 70 cGy/fr; (3) right lateral : 30 cGy/fr; (4) left lateral: 30 cGy/fr.

5.7.2 Radical post-pneumonectomy radiotherapy

This is performed 4–6 weeks after a radical surgery in cases of high risk of recurrence (node involvement or positive margin of resection). The target volume is the mediastinum, the resection and the supraclavicular nodes. The prescribed dose is 50 Gy. The technique is a three-field technique with wedges and 18 MV linear accelerator.

- *Position.* Supine with the arms raised on the head.
- *Mediastinum field margins.*
  Anterior and posterior field:

  upper limit: joint with the supraclavicular field

lower limit: about 4 cm below the carina
lateral limits: 1 cm of the vertebral bodies on the opposite side
of the resection, 3 cm of the resection on the side of surgery.

Lateral field:

upper and lower limits: as above
anterior limit: 3 cm in front of the trachea
posterior limit: 3 cm behind the trachea.

- *Beam modifications.* Block on AP–PA fields.
- *Dose prescription* (Figure 5.5). The total dose at the axis intersection is 50 Gy in 25 fractions over 5 weeks.

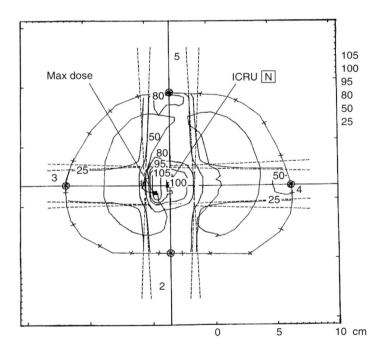

Figure 5.4 Radical irradiation with rotation therapy. Isodose distribution
for cobalt and SSD = 80 cm. [N] normalized on the 100% (ICRU) point;
(■) maximum dose 109%. Loading: (1) anterior: 70 cGy/fr; (2) posterior:
70 cGy/fr; (3) right lateral: 30 cGy/fr; (4) left lateral: 30 cGy/fr; (5)
cyclotherapy: 200 cGy/fr.

5.7.3 Palliative radiotherapy

This is used to palliate symptoms such as haemoptysis in cases of large tumour or metastasis. The target volume is restricted to the tumour of the lung. The prescribed dose is 30 Gy which is given with an accelerated regimen. The technique involves two parallel AP–PA fields with telecobalt.

- *Position.* Supine.
- *Field margins.* Anterior and posterior field limits: about 2 or 3 cm around the tumour.
- *Dose prescription.* The dose used is 30 Gy in 10 fractions, five fractions per week.

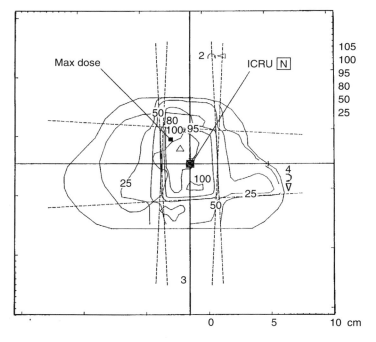

Figure 5.5 Post-pneumonectomy irradiation. Isodose distribution for 18 MV and SAD. N normalized on the 100% (ICRU) point; (■) maximum dose 104%. Loading: (1, 2) anterior: 100 cGy/fr; (3) posterior: 45 cGy/fr; (4) left lateral: 55 cGy/fr.

Table 5.2 Chemotherapy combinations for small-cell carcinoma of the lung

Acronym	Drug combination
COPP–CCNU	Cyclophosphamide (endoxan)
	Vincristine (oncovin)
	CCNU (belustine)
	Procarbazin (natulan)
CEV	Cyclophosphamide
	Epirubin (adriamycin)
	Vincristine
EVC-VP-16	Epirubin
	Vincristine
	Cyclophosphamide
	VP–16 (etoposide)
CDDP–VP–16	CDD platinum (cisplatyl)
	Methylprednisolone
	VP–16
Endoxan–VP–16	Cyclophosphamide
	VP–16

Table 5.3 Chemotherapy combinations for non-small-cell carcinoma of the lung

Acronym	Drug combination
COM	Cyclophosphamide
	Vincristine
	MTX
CE	*Cis*-platinum
	Epirubicin
Carboplatinum	Carboplatinum (paraplatin)
Carboplatinum + VP–16	Carboplatinum
(C–E)	VP–16 (etoposide)

5.8 MORBIDITY

Radiation transverse myelitis is a major risk and every effort must be made to keep the spinal cord dose below the dangerous level of 35 Gy in 17 days or its equivalent (45–50 Gy at dose rates of 200 to 180 cGy per fraction respectively). Severe symptomatic pulmonary fibrosis should not occur in more than 5% of patients receiving up to 60 Gy. This condition is invariably preceded by an attack of acute radiation pneumonitis occurring 6 to 12 weeks after treatment.

Fibrotic pneumonitis is associated with pre-existing chronic bronchitis, chemotherapeutic agents such as bleomycin, and too extensive target volumes.

5.9 CHEMOTHERAPY

Tables 5.2 and 5.3 give the combinations of chemotherapy for small-cell carcinoma of the lung and non-small cell carcinoma of the lung.

6

Breast

6.1 INCIDENCE AND RISK FACTORS

The risk factors for breast cancer are usually associated with endocrine, metabolic and genetic factors. They include patients > 50 years old, history of early menarche, late natural menopause, nulliparity and age at first full-term pregnancy (increased risk in patients who had their first child after the age of 30), and a family history of breast cancer. Other factors that may increase the risk for breast cancer include exposure to ionizing irradiation and total dietary fat.

6.2 PRESENTATION AND NATURAL HISTORY

It is now recognized that carcinoma of the breast originates in the secreting unit of the breast. As the tumour grows, it spreads through the breast by direct infiltration, along mammary ducts, and by breast lymphatics.

The appearance of a palpable mass is the most common presenting sign. The upper left or right quadrant is the most common site of origin and approximately 50–60% of women have tumours larger than 2 cm in diameter at presentation. Other signs and symptoms of breast cancer include pain in the breast (6%), nipple discharge (4.5%), nipple retraction (3%), skin dimpling (3%), nipple erosion (2%), axillary tumour (1.5%), skin oedema (1.5%), skin erythema (1.5%) and breast enlargement (1%). Some patients will present with more than one sign or symptom. Occasionally, axillary lymphadenopathy may be the presenting finding. Approximately 10% of patients will have distant metastases at presentation. Simultaneous bilateral breast cancer is a rare event (1–2%).

Breast cancers may progress locally, regionally and distantly. Locally, the tumour may grow into the superficial or deep lymphatics and produce oedema of the skin (peau d'orange). If the tumour is left untreated, ulceration of the skin may develop. This can be associated with skin fixation over the tumour and localized erythema. As the cancer progresses locally, the ulceration may enlarge to a massive fungating, foul-smelling mass. Satellite nodules in the skin over the breast are a sign of widespread disease within the breast.

Breast cancer frequently metastasizes to regional lymph nodes with the axillary nodes generally being the first to be involved. Approximately 20% of patients with T1 lesions and 45% of patients with T2 lesions will have metastases to axillary nodes at presentation. The frequency of axillary lymph node metastases also varies with the site of the tumour in the breast and it is more frequent from primary tumours in the upper outer quadrant.

Lymph node involvement in the internal mammary and supraclavicular areas may also occur but is less common than axillary metastases. The incidence of metastatic involvement of the internal mammary lymphatic chain correlates with the location of the primary tumour and the presence or absence of axillary node metastases. Patients with tumours in the upper outer quadrant and negative axillary nodes have a low incidence of metastatic disease (2–5%), whereas the incidence is about 50% in those with inner quadrant lesions and positive nodes in the axilla. Metastases to supraclavicular nodes are related to the stage of the disease and the status of the axillary and internal mammary nodes. However, less than 5% of patients will present with palpable disease. In surgical series, the incidence of supraclavicular lymphatic metastasis ranges from 2–6% for patients with negative axillary and internal mammary nodes to 17–43% for patients with axillary and parasternal nodal involvement.

Haematogenous spread may be observed even with small tumours. The most common sites for metastases from breast cancer are the lung, bone, liver, adrenal gland, kidney, ovaries and brain.

6.3 HISTOPATHOLOGY

A number of pathological classifications of breast cancer are currently used. Table 6.1 outlines the classification recommended by

Table 6.1 Modified WHO pathological classification of cancer of the breast

Stage	Description
1	*Carcinoma*
A	Intraductal and intralobular non-infiltrating carcinoma
B	Infiltrating ductal carcinoma
C	Special histological variants of carcinoma
1	Medullary carcinoma
2	Papillary carcinoma
3	Cribriform carcinoma
4	Mucous carcinoma
5	Lobular carcinoma
6	Squamous cell carcinoma
7	Paget's disease of the breast
8	Carcinoma arising in cellular intracanicular fibroadenoma
2	*Sarcoma*
3	*Carcinosarcoma*
4	*Unclassified tumour*

the World Health Organization. Infiltrating ductal carcinoma, not otherwise specified, is by far the most common tumour. Other types of carcinomas that arise from large ducts include medullary, papillary, lobular, mucinous, tubular, etc.

6.4 INVESTIGATIONS

The evaluation of any patient with breast cancer must begin with a complete history and physical examination. Menstrual status, parity and family history of cancer should be noted. The entire breast should be examined and any change recorded. Careful examination of the adjacent lymph node-bearing areas must be performed. Abdominal and pelvic examinations are essential.

Laboratory studies should include a complete blood count and an alkaline phosphatase test. A chest radiograph should be performed. In an asymptomatic patient with early stage disease (stages I and II) and a normal alkaline phosphatase test, bone and liver scans should not be routinely performed. If possible, oestrogen and progesterone receptors should be assayed as both have therapeutic implications and predictive prognostic value. Recently, flow cytometry and the thymidine-labelling index have been used to measure the growth fraction of tumours and can also be used as prognostic indicators.

Table 6.2 Staging classification for breast cancer (UICC, 1987)

Stage		Description
T		Primary tumour
TX		Primary tumour cannot be assessed
T0		No evidence of primary tumour
Tis		Carcinoma *in situ*: intraductal carcinoma or lobular carcinoma *in situ* or Paget's disease of the nipple with no tumour
T1		Tumour 2 cm or less in greatest dimension
	T1a	0.5 cm or less in greatest dimension
	T1b	More than 0.5 cm but no more than 1 cm in greatest dimension
	T1c	More than 1 cm but no more than 2 cm in greatest dimension
T2		Tumour more than 2 cm but no more than 5 cm in greatest dimension
T3		Tumour more than 5 cm in greatest dimension
T4		Tumour of any size with direct extension to chest wall or skin
	T4a	Extension to chest wall
	T4b	Oedema (including peau d'orange) or ulceration of the skin or satellite skin nodules confined to the same breast
	T4c	Both 4a *and* 4b, above
	T4d	Inflammatory carcinoma
N		Regional lymph node metastasis
NX		Regional lymph nodes cannot be assessed
N0		No regional lymph node metastasis
N1		Metastasis to moveable ipsilateral axillary node(s)
N2		Metastasis to ipsilateral axillary node(s) fixed to one another or to other structures
N3		Metastasis to ipsilateral internal mammary lymph node(s)
M		Distant metastasis
MX		Presence of distant metastasis cannot be assessed
M0		No distant metastasis
M1		Distant metastasis (includes metastasis to supraclavicular lymph nodes)

6.5 STAGING AND PROGNOSIS

There are few staging classifications available. The UICC staging classification, outlined in Tables 6.2 and 6.3, is the most frequently used and is the one we recommend.

There is marked variability in the clinical course of patients with breast cancer. Some women with small tumours die of metastatic

Table 6.3 Stage grouping (UICC, 1987)

Stage	T	N	M
0	Tis	N0	M0
I	T1	N0	M0
IIA	T0	N1	M0
	T1	N1	M0
	T2	N0	M0
IIB	T2	N1	M0
	T3	N0	M0
IIIA	T0	N2	M0
	T1	N2	M0
	T2	N2	M0
	T3	N1, N2	M0
IIIB	T4	Any N	M0
	Any T	N3	M0
IV	Any T	Any N	M1

disease within months, whereas others with more advanced lesions survive for several decades without any evidence of disease progression. Identifying possible prognostic factors that might predict tumour behaviour is important because different therapeutic approaches can be designed based on these variables.

Tumour size is an established prognostic factor in breast cancer with larger tumours being associated with shorter intervals before disease recurrence and/or death. There is a direct relationship between the size of the tumour and incidence of local recurrence. In tumours less than 1 cm in diameter, the probability of relapse is approximately 10%, compared to 25% for patients with tumours between 1 and 2 cm in diameter.

Axillary node metastasis is also an important prognostic factor both for local recurrence and survival. Node-negative patients have a much lower disease recurrence than node-positive patients (6% compared with 25%). Survival is also affected by metastatic involvement of the axillary nodes. Women without disease in the nodes have a 20% greater chance of five-year survival than those with positive nodes, for tumours of similar size. The total number of nodes involved is also important. Patients with four or more positive lymph nodes have a diminished survival, compared to those with fewer involved nodes.

Histopathological characteristics of the tumour are associated with biological tumour behaviour. Several histological features such

Table 6.4 Survival rates (%) for different stages of breast cancer

Stage	Five-year survival	Ten-year survival
I	70–95	60–80
II	50–80	40–60
III	10–50	0–30
IV	0–10	0–5

as degree of cellular differentiation, mitotic rate and nuclear anaplasia correlate with a poor outcome.

Hormonal receptors have an important predictive prognostic value. Patients with negative or low hormonal receptor levels (oestrogen and progesterone) have a higher recurrence rate and shorter overall survival than patients with positive measurements. Flow cytometry and the thymidine-labelling index, which assess the growth characteristics of a tumour, have been shown to be of prognostic importance. The difficulties in performing the techniques may prevent these becoming widely available for clinical use.

Table 6.4 summarizes the treatment results, by stage, for patients with breast cancer. Factors other than stage, including tumour histology and grade, age, tumour growth rate, etc., have been shown to influence prognosis and they must be taken into account when individual patients are being assessed. The number of positive axillary nodes appears to be the single most important predictor of survival. The ten-year survival rate for node-negative patients is approximately 75% compared with 25% for those with positive nodes. In patients with three or fewer positive nodes, the ten-year survival rate is about 35%, decreasing to about 15% for patients with four or more positive axillary nodes.

6.6 TREATMENT – CHOICE OF MODALITY

6.6.1 Radical treatment

Breast cancer is a typical pathology in which a multidisciplinary team approach is essential to obtain the best clinical outcome. Close interaction among the various specialities including the surgeon, the radiation oncologist and the medical oncologist is of utmost importance. Only a few patients with breast cancer will not require the active participation of each of these professionals during the course of their disease management.

Surgery plays a major role in the diagnosis and treatment of breast cancer. Over the years, many surgical procedures have been introduced in the management of this disease, including radical mastectomy, super-radical mastectomy, modified radical mastectomy, simple mastectomy, and segmentectomy or tumourectomy. Segmental mastectomy (quadrantectomy) followed by local radiotherapy is now an accepted and recommended therapeutic approach to the treatment of patients with T1 and T2 disease, having the advantage of preserving the breast and yet achieving local control similar to that of the most mutilating surgical procedure. A more radical procedure, such as the modified radical mastectomy, should be reserved for patients with lesions larger than 5 cm in diameter, and patients with small breasts in whom tumourectomy would lead to a poor cosmetic result. If possible, an axillary dissection involving levels I and II should always be carried out for all patients undergoing surgery, regardless of the tumour size, stage or surgical technique.

The role of radiotherapy in improving local disease control has been well established in many retrospective and prospective studies. Like surgery, radiotherapy is a local treatment modality. There is no need to irradiate the axilla in most of the patients who have undergone a full axillary dissection. Lymphatic irradiation should be reserved for patients with massive axillary infiltration by metastatic disease, for patients with gross residual disease left behind, or for patients in whom the tumour has spread through the capsule of the node into the axillary fat. For those patients in whom a radical mastectomy has been performed, chest wall radiotherapy is only indicated if patients have high-risk factors for local recurrence, such as large primary lesions (> 5 cm in diameter), vascular–lymphatic space invasion, skin or muscle invasion, and multicentric disease. Radiotherapy is also frequently employed in the palliative treatment of patients with metastatic disease.

Chemotherapy, once used only for metastatic or locally advanced disease, is now frequently employed as an adjunct to the primary breast treatment. It is now commonly believed that breast cancer is often a systemic disease at diagnosis and therefore no longer curable by local therapy alone. Systemic drugs are used in an effort to eradicate cancer cells remaining after primary local treatment. A Consensus Development Committee convened by the National

Cancer Institute in the USA made the following recommendations regarding adjuvant systemic therapy:

- premenopausal women with positive axillary nodes should receive adjuvant systemic chemotherapy;
- premenopausal women with negative axillary nodes should be considered for adjuvant chemotherapy if they are felt to be at high risk for recurrence (high degree of differentiation, negative for receptors, large tumours, etc.);
- postmenopausal women with positive nodes and positive hormone receptor levels should receive tamoxifen;
- postmenopausal women with positive axillary nodes and negative hormone receptor levels should not receive adjuvant chemotherapy routinely but rather be assessed on an individual basis; and
- postmenopausal women with negative axillary nodes do not need adjuvant chemotherapy.

Table 6.5 shows the most frequently used chemotherapy combinations.

Hormone therapy has an important role in the management of metastatic disease. The routine adjuvant use of endocrine therapy should be reserved for postmenopausal patients with positive nodes and positive hormonal receptor levels. For premenopausal women, its benefit remains unproven. Bilateral oophorectomy (ovarian cas-

Table 6.5 Commonly used combination chemotherapy programmes

Regimen	Drugs used
CMF	Cyclophosphamide
	Methotrexate
	5-fluorouracil
FAC	5-fluorouracil
	Adriamycin
	Cyclophosphamide
'COOPER'	Cyclophosphamide
	Methotrexate
	5-fluorouracil
	Vincristine
	Prednisone
CAMF	Cyclophosphamide
	Adriamycin
	Methotrexate
	5-fluorouracil

tration) and hypophysectomy–adrenalectomy are rarely used now. Oestrogen therapy (diethylstilboestrol 5 mg three times a day) was frequently used in the past. However, it was associated with many side-effects and its use has been almost completely abandoned. Other hormonal therapies that are infrequently utilized include androgens (testosterone propionate 100 mg intramuscularly three times a week or fluoxymesterone 10 mg by mouth twice a day) and progestational agents (medroxyprogesterone 100 mg intramuscularly three times a week). Recently, the anti-oestrogen tamoxifen (20 mg twice a day) has generally replaced all other agents in the hormonal management of patients with breast cancer.

6.6.2 Pallative treatment

Patients with locally advanced breast cancer may include those with large operable tumours or those considered inoperable but without distant metastases. These patients usually have a poor prognosis, including those with T3N0 disease. Combination chemotherapy should be used either before or after local treatment. For inoperable tumours, irradiation improves local control, but doses of 70 Gy or higher must be delivered. Increasing doses of irradiation will result in more severe complications, including a 5% incidence of brachial plexus injury. Inoperable tumours may become operable after a dose of 50 Gy.

Fungating tumour masses in conjunction with diffuse metastatic disease may be treated with a hypofractionated regimen delivering either 20 Gy in 5 fractions or 30 Gy in 10 fractions to the chest wall, peripheral lymphatic system and axilla, depending on disease extension, using techniques applied in definitive treatment.

In the supraclavicular and axillary areas, further external beam irradiation is often necessary for palliation. Superficial hyperthermia is often administered with external beam irradiation in attempts to augment tumour regression. Risks involved with re-irradiation include severe fibrosis and necrosis of soft tissue and bone, and brachial plexopathy. However, the therapeutic balance between necessary palliation of often debilitating symptoms and potential risk for complications must be considered. Patients with an overall poor prognosis may benefit from short-term palliation of symptoms and not survive long enough to experience late complications of re-irradiation.

6.7 RADIOTHERAPY TECHNIQUE

6.7.1 Treatment of the intact breast

This is performed 3–5 weeks after conservative surgery. The target volume includes the entire breast. The prescribed dose is 50 Gy to the target volume. A boost dose can be delivered on the tumour bed either by interstitial implant or electron beam. The technique involves two tangentially directed fields with telecobalt.

- *Position*. Supine with the arm carefully immobilized in an abducted position.
- *Localization*. Marks on breast scar.
- *Field margins* (Figures 6.1 and 6.2).
  The field size is 16–18 cm × 7–9 cm:

  > medial limit: midline of the patient along the mid-sternal line
  > lateral limit: 2 cm lateral to the palpable breast tissue, usually along the mid-axillary line
  > superior limit: level of the sternoclavicular joint (angle of Louis); if needed, the border may be moved superiorly to include the entire breast
  > inferior limit: 2 cm below the inframammary fold

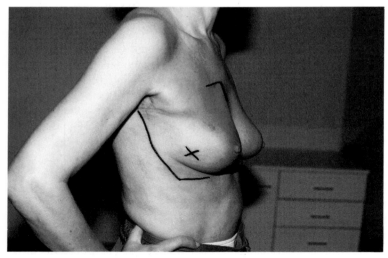

Figure 6.1 Irradiation after conservative surgery. Skin marks.

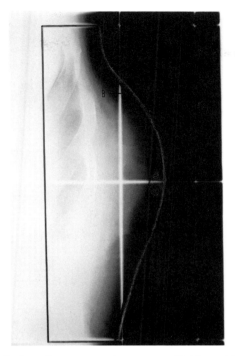

Figure 6.2 Irradiation after conservative surgery. Outline of the field limits on a radiograph. B, limit of the breast.

- *Beam modifications.* The contour is obtained at the midline axis. Compensating wedge filters (usually of 45°) must be used so that a homogeneous dose distribution is achieved within the treated volume.
- *Dose prescription* (Figure 6.3). The total dose at the midline axis is 50 Gy in 25 fractions over 5 weeks.

6.7.2 Treatment of the supraclavicular and axillary nodes

The supraclavicular and apical axillary nodes are irradiated when there is an axilla lymph node involvement. The entire axilla is only irradiated when there is massive axilla lymph node involvement and/or extracapsular node involvement. The prescribed dose is 50 Gy to these volumes. The technique involves an anterior field with telecobalt angled 10–12° to the ipsilateral side so that irradia-

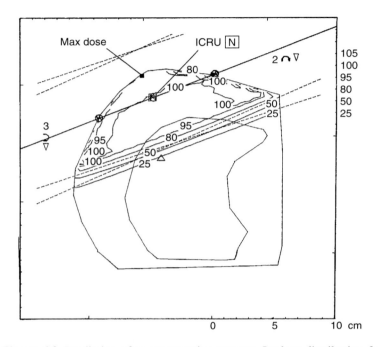

Figure 6.3 Irradiation after conservative surgery. Isodose distribution for cobalt and SSD = 80 cm. N normalized on the 100% (ICRU) point. (■) maximum dose 104%. Loading: (1,3) external tangential: 100 cGy/fr; (2, 4) internal tangential: 100 cGy/fr.

tion of the trachea and oesophagus is avoided. A posterior axillary field with telecobalt is employed to supplement the dose to the midplane of the axilla. The midline dose is calculated at the mid-separation between the anterior and posterior axillary surfaces at the central axis of the posterior axillary boost.

- *Position.* Supine with the arm in an abducted position.
- *Field margins.*
  Anterior axilla and supraclavicular:

    lower limit: coincides with the superior limit of the tangential
    field at the level of the angle of Louis
    medial limit: midline of the patient
    superior limit: at the level of the cricothyroid groove

lateral limit: medial aspect of the humeral head – when the entire axilla is to be included, the lateral border should be extended to include the lateral aspect of the humeral head which should be shielded

Posterior axilla:

medial limit: 1 cm inside a parallel to the thoracic cage
superior limit: superior aspect of the clavicle
lateral limit: lateral aspect of the humeral head
inferior limit: same level as superior border of tangential fields

- *Dose prescription.* The dose to the anterior field is prescribed at the maximum, taking care not to give the anterior axilla more than 65 Gy. The dose from the posterior axillar field is calculated so that the midplane of the axilla receives a total dose of 50 Gy in 25 fractions over 5 weeks.

6.8 MORBIDITY

Surgical complications are usually only seen following radical procedures and include arm oedema, skin flap necrosis, haematoma, wound dehiscence and infection. Problems of psychological and social adjustment to mastectomy are observed in about 50% of the patients.

Radiotherapy is usually well tolerated. Acute toxicities are self-limited and consist mostly of skin changes (erythema, moist desqua-mation). Late complications include breast oedema/fibrosis, arm oedema in 5–7% of cases, and asymptomatic lung fibrosis. For patients undergoing breast-conserving surgery plus radiotherapy, mild to moderate radiation sequelae will occur in approximately 25% of the patients. Severe sequelae are expected to occur in less than 1% of cases and are clearly dose dependent. Brachial plexo-pathy, breast necrosis, rib fracture, pneumonitis and transient pleural effusion are rare complications occurring in less than 1% of cases.

Chemotherapy can be very toxic and should only be delivered under expert supervision. The most common acute side-effects include nausea and vomiting, leucopenia and thrombocytopenia which can increase susceptibility to infections and haemorrhage, mucositis, alopecia and renal failure. Late toxicity may involve the cardiovascular, nervous, respiratory and renal systems.

6.9 SPECIAL CONSIDERATIONS

6.9.1 Lobular carcinoma *in situ*

The true incidence of lobular carcinoma is not known, but is thought to range from 0.8% to 3.6% of all benign epithelial breast lesions. Approximately 20–30% of patients with lobular carcinoma *in situ* will go on to develop invasive cancer of various histological types. There is no consensus on the optimal treatment. Observation has gradually been accepted as the treatment of choice, although some authors recommend unilateral mastectomy plus mirror biopsy of the contralateral breast. Radiotherapy does not appear to have any role in the management of this disease.

6.9.2 Inflammatory breast cancer

Inflammatory breast cancer accounts for 1–4% of breast cancers. The diagnosis is usually made on clinical–pathological grounds. The clinical features include erythema and oedema of the breast, frequently without an associated mass. The typical histological finding is dermal lymphatic invasion with tumour. Inflammatory breast cancer carries an ominous prognosis and it should be treated as a systemic disease. Surgery alone is contra-indicated because of a very high local relapse rate and poor survival. The current therapeutic recommendation is maximum doses of systemic therapy with a doxorubicin-containing regimen. Radiation and surgery may be used after chemotherapy to decrease the recurrence rate.

6.9.3 Bilateral breast cancer

Bilateral breast cancers can present as synchronous or meta-chronous events. The majority are metachronous. The incidence of synchronous bilateral cancer is approximately 1–2% of bilateral cancers. Prognosis is dependent on the stage of the disease and the treatment should be that appropriate for the stage of the disease.

6.9.4 Cystosarcoma phylloides

This tumour is the most common of the non-epithelial lesions of the breast. Surgery is the treatment of choice with less than 5% of patients with benign tumours experiencing recurrence. The incidence of positive axillary adenopathy is low. Radiotherapy has no role in the management of these tumours, except in patients with residual, recurrent or inoperable tumours.

6.9.5 Male breast cancer

Male breast cancer is uncommon and constitutes only 1% of all breast cancers and less than 1% of all malignant tumours in men. The pathological types are similar to those found in women, except that lobular carcinoma *in situ* does not occur in men. There is no consensus for loco-regional management. The standard local treatment is a mastectomy with or without post-operative radiotherapy. The role of adjuvant hormonal therapy or chemotherapy is unclear. Ten-year survival rates are 70%, 45% and 10% for stages I, II and III, respectively.

7

Rectum

7.1 INCIDENCE AND RISK FACTORS

Cancer of the rectum is more common in industrialized countries. A low intake of meat and lipids, and a diet rich in fibre, vegetables and fresh fruits may be a good method of primary prevention of rectal cancer. The incidence rate (standardized for the world population) is around 12/100 000 in industrialized countries and 5/100 000 in developing countries. Rectal cancer is slightly more frequent in men than in women and represents 30% of tumours arising in the large bowel.

Familial risk factors include familial polyposis, association with cancer of the breast, endometrium or ovary and familial cancer of the rectum. Personal risk factors include previous treatment for cancer of the colon, benign adenomatous polyp and villous polyp, ulcerative colitis and Crohn's disease.

7.2 PRESENTATION AND NATURAL HISTORY

Blood in the stools is the most frequent presenting symptom. At an advanced stage, occlusion, pelvic or perineal abcesses or distant metastases may be the first signs, with alteration of general health.

At an early stage, cancer of the rectum presents as a polypoid tumour of length 2–3 cm, which then becomes ulcerated and tends to become circular and penetrate through the rectal wall into the peri-rectal fat and surrounding tissue (vagina and uterus in women, prostate in men, bladder ureter, lateral and posterior pelvic walls). The peri-rectal nodes are often invaded, and then the cancer cells proceed through the lymphatic channels to the origin of the inferior mesenteric vein at the level of S3 and then along these vessels to the paraortic region. The most frequent site of metastasis is the liver, more rarely the lung, brain, bones or subclavian nodes.

7.3 HISTOPATHOLOGY

In most cases, the pathological report on the biopsy will indicate an adenocarcinoma of Lieberkuhnian type that is well or moderately differentiated. Colloid aspects may be present, and both these and undifferentiated type carry a poorer prognosis. Lymphomas and epidermoid or carcinoid tumours are rare.

7.4 INVESTIGATIONS

The diagnosis can very often be done by a careful rectal examination which is also one of the best means to appreciate the local extension of the tumour and its resectability. Rectoscopy is mandatory to see the tumour and perform a biopsy. Barium enemas give a good idea of the endoluminal extension. Sonography or computed tomographic scan may be performed, if available, to assess the primary tumour, the presence of paraortic nodes, and, most importantly, liver metastases. The carcino-embryonic antigen level is usually correlated with the extent of the tumour.

7.5 STAGING AND PROGNOSIS

There are different classifications of post-operative stage, of which the first was the original Dukes categories (A, B and C; Dukes, 1932). There is no widely used pre-therapeutic classification. The clinical TNM–UICC classification (1987) is identical to the pathological (post-surgical) classification (Table 7.1).

External irradiation in association with surgery has been shown to reduce the rate of pelvic relapse but any improvement in cure rate is still controversial, as is the relevance of pre- versus post-operative irradiation even though pre-operative radiotherapy seems more efficient locally than post-operative irradiation, in recent randomized trials.

When it is not possible to eradicate by surgery all gross tumour because it is fixed to the pelvis or because of extension to the

Table 7.1 Classifications of rectal cancer

Classification	Stage	Description
Dukes (1932)	A	Tumour confined to rectal wall
	B	Extension to peri-rectal fat or through the serosa
	C	Any tumour with lymph node involvement
TNM	T1	Tumour confined to mucosa or submucosa
(UICC, 1987)	T2	Extension to muscularis propria but not through the rectal wall
	T3	Extension to peri-rectal fat or through the serosa
	T4	Tumour with adhesion to surrounding structures
	N0	No lymphatic involvement
	N1	Extension to 1–3 lymph nodes
	N2	Extension to 4 or more lymph nodes

Table 7.2 Results of treatment of rectal cancer

Stage	Local pelvic relapse after radical surgery alone (%)	Five-year overall survival after radical treatment (%)
pT1 N0	< 5	90
pT2 N0	10	70–80
pT3 N0	15–20	60
pT4 N0	30–40	40
pT1 T2 N1	15–20	60
pT3 N1 N2	30	30–40
pT4 N1 N2	40–60	5–20
Pelvic recurrence after radical surgery		5
Solitary liver metastases with complete resection		0–20

paraortic nodes or diffuse metastases to the liver or other organs, only palliation can be offered to the patient. Relief of pain and haemorrhagic discharge should be the objective with an average survival of 6–12 months but also some long-term survivals of two or three or more years. Table 7.2 gives the average survival according to different stages and treatments.

7.6 TREATMENT – CHOICE OF MODALITY

7.6.1 Radical treatment

Surgery is the basic treatment of rectal cancer. When presenting with occlusion or perforation and infection, cancer of the rectum is usually treated with a primary diverting colostomy. Curative treatment is performed at a second stage whenever possible.

Generally, external irradiation is used in conjunction with surgery to improve the local control in the pelvis. Chemotherapy with a regimen containing 5-fluorouracil is still being researched as a curative treatment. When a large tumour is fixed to the pelvis, preoperative irradiation is sometimes beneficial to shrink the tumour and give a chance of curative resection. In some selected cases, resection of a liver metastasis may lead to long-term survival and sometimes cure.

7.6.2 Palliative treatment

When surgery cannot be performed for T3–T4 cancers or pelvic recurrences, cure is usually impossible. Diverting colostomy is recommended for obstruction, incontinence or distressing bloody discharge.

The therapeutic approach for locally advanced carcinoma of the rectum again gives priority to the need to achieve durable symptomatic control given the difficulty in effectively relieving pain associated with bowel obstruction and invasion of the sacral plexus. To achieve this, clinical data support the administration of conventional irradiation to patients with disease localized to the pelvis rather than a more abbreviated course of therapy. Inoperable patients without a prior history of irradiation and with extensive disease and associated symptoms can be palliated by delivering 30 Gy in 10 fractions or 35 Gy in 14 fractions to the pelvis.

7.7 RADIOTHERAPY TECHNIQUES

7.7.1 Radical post-operative irradiation

This is performed 4–6 weeks after radical surgery in cases of high risk of recurrence in the posterior part of the pelvis (p T3, T4, N1,

N2). The target volume is the posterior pelvis. The prescribed dose is 50 Gy to this volume.

The technique is a four-field box technique with telecobalt.

- *Position.* Prone with a fully distended bladder.
- *Localization.* Marks on perineal scar, anal margin and/or vagina.
- *Field margins.*
  Posterior and anterior fields (12 × 10 cm to 18 × 13 cm):

  > upper limit: low rectum: S1–S2; upper rectum: L5–S1
  > lower limit: after Miles' amputation: lower extremity of perineal scar; after anterior resection: 4 cm below the anastomosis
  > lateral limits: pelvic rim

  Lateral field (12 × 9 cm to 18 × 12 cm):

  > upper and lower limits: as above
  > posterior limit: 2 cm behind the anterior bony sacral margin
  > anterior limit: 1 cm anterior to the promontory of the sacrum (may vary according to anatomy of the patients and location of the tumour)

- *Beam modifications.* Blocks on AP–PA fields.
- *Dose prescription* (Figure 7.1). The total dose at the axis intersection is 50 Gy in 25 fractions over 5 weeks.
- *Special consideration.* It is possible to add 10 Gy on a reduced boost field of 7 × 7 cm, especially if the target volume has been demarcated by clips and no small bowel is included in the field.

7.7.2 Radical pre-operative irradiation

Surgery is usually performed 4 weeks after the end of radiotherapy. The target volume includes tumour and the posterior pelvis. The prescribed dose is 46 Gy to this volume. The technique is a three-field technique with wedges and an 18 MV linear accelerator.

- *Position.* Prone with a fully distended bladder.
- *Localization.* Rectum filled with barium enema; marks on the anal margin.
- *Field margins* (Figures 7.2 and 7.3).
  Posterior field (12 × 10 cm to 16 × 13 cm):

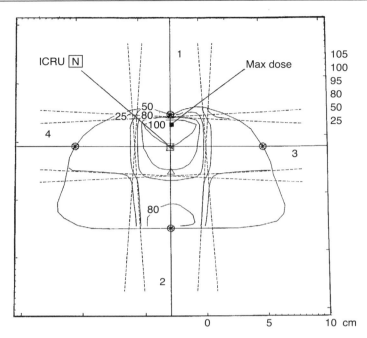

Figure 7.1 Post-operative irradiation. Isodose distribution for cobalt and SSD = 80 cm. ⒩ normalized on the 100% (ICRU) point; (■) maximum dose 104%. Loading: (1) posterior: 80 cGy/fr; (2) anterior: 60 cGy/fr; (3) right lateral: 30 cGy/fr; (4) left lateral: 30 cGy/fr.

upper limit: low rectum: S1–S2; upper rectum: L5–S1
lower limit: 4 cm below the lower end of the tumour or at the anal margin
lateral limits: pelvic rim

Lateral fields (12 × 19 cm to 16 × 12 cm):

upper and lower limits: as above
posterior limit: 2 cm behind the anterior bony sacral margin
anterior limit: 1 cm anterior to the promontorium of the sacrum (may vary according to anatomy of the patients and location of the tumour but should be at least 3 cm anterior to the tumour)

● *Beam modifications.* Wedges of 45° must be positioned in the lateral fields at each session.

- *Dose prescription* (Figure 7.4). The total dose at the axis intersection is 46 Gy in 23 fractions over 4½ weeks.
- *Special consideration.* It is possible to use an accelerated irradiation giving 36 Gy in 12 fractions of 3 Gy over 17 days (5

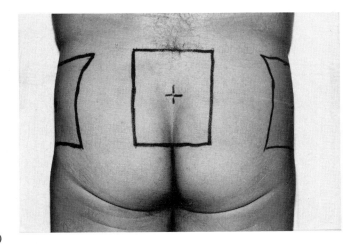

(a)

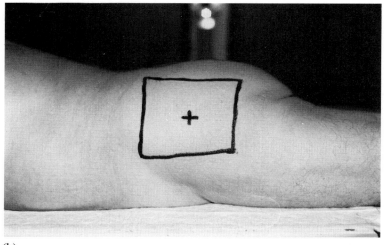

(b)

Figure 7.2 Radical pre-operative irradiation. Skin marks: (a) posterior field; (b) lateral field.

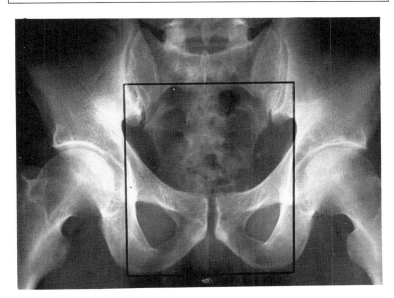

(a)

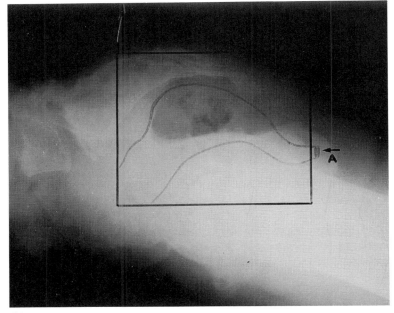

(b)

Figure 7.3 Radical pre-operative irradiation. Outline of the field limits on a radiograph: (a) posterior field; (b) lateral field. Posterior limit is tangential to the posterior part of the sacral bone. A, anal margin.

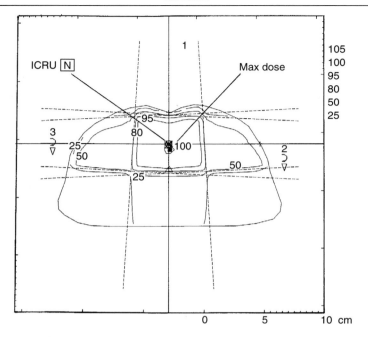

Figure 7.4 Pre-operative irradiation. Isodose distribution for 18 MV X-rays and SAD = 100 cm. ⃞N normalized on the 100% (ICRU) point; (■) maximum dose 104%. Loading: (1) posterior: 100 cGy/fr; (2) right lateral: 50 cGy/fr; (3) left lateral: 50 cGy/fr.

fractions per week) or 25 Gy in 5 fractions of 5 Gy over 5 days. Whenever possible, irradiation to such deeply sited target volumes should be given with beams of 10–20 MV.

7.7.3 Palliative irradiation

This is performed for large fixed non-resectable (T4) tumours, for T3 tumours in fragile inoperable patients or for pelvic recurrences. The target volume is restricted to the detectable tumour in the pelvis. It does not include all the potential subclinical extension of the tumour. The prescribed dose is 40–45 Gy, which is usually given with an accelerated regimen. The technique is two parallel AP–PA fields with telecobalt.

- *Position.* Prone with the buttocks taped apart to avoid moist desquamation in the buttock sulcus.

- *Localization.* Marks on the anal margin.
- *Field margins.*
  Anterior and posterior fields (12×10 cm to 16×13 cm):

    upper limit: lower rectum: S1–S2: upper rectum: L5–S1
    lower limit: 4 cm below the lower end of the tumour or at the
    anal margin
    lateral limits: pelvic rim

- *Dose prescription* (Figure 7.5). The total dose at the axis is 30 Gy
  in 10 fractions over 2 weeks.
- *Special consideration.* In cases of good regression and good
  tolerance, a second course of 12 Gy in 4 fractions of 3 Gy can be
  given 4–6 weeks later. If the anteroposterior diameter of the
  patient exceeds 20 cm a four-field box technique should be used
  to avoid overdosage of superficial tissues.

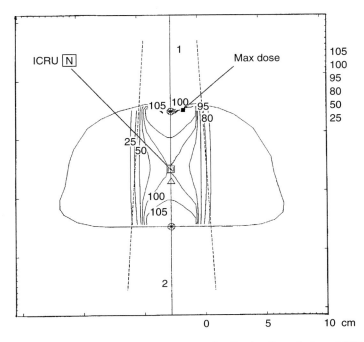

Figure 7.5 Palliative irradiation. Isodose distribution for cobalt and SSD =
80 cm. [N] normalized on the 100% (ICRU) point; (■) maximum dose
112%. Loading: (1) posterior: 150 cGy/fr; (2) anterior: 150 cGy/fr.

7.8 MORBIDITY

Irradiation of the pelvis can lead to acute side-effects such as cystitis, proctitis, ileitis or epidermitis which may require symptomatic treatment. Pre-operative irradiation delays perineal wound healing after Miles' operation but does not increase the risk of anastomotic leakage after anterior resection. Late complications are mainly ileal radiation injury in cases of post-operative radiotherapy.

8

Liver

8.1 INCIDENCE AND RISK FACTORS

Liver cancer is one of the most serious tumours in China, with an annual mortality rate of 10/100 000. It ranks third following gastric and oesophageal cancers. The highest incidence appears to be in West Africa (higher than 50/100 000). The age range is from 25 to 60, with an average of 45 years. The male:female ratio is about 4:1. In France, the incidence is about 4/100 000, at the same level as pancreatic cancer, while in China the hepatic:pancreatic ratio is about 8:1.

Possible carcinogenic factors for hepatic cancer include hepatitis B type virus, aflatoxin in mildewed peanuts, and alcoholic cirrhosis of the liver.

8.2 PRESENTATION AND NATURAL HISTORY

The patient usually has right upper abdominal pain, and is asthenic with fatigue and weight loss.

The liver may or may not be enlarged, depending on the size of the tumour, which may be hard and/or painful. Multiple tumour masses can often make irregularities of the liver surface.

All patients with cirrhosis of liver must be followed up carefully, because cirrhotic livers may harbour one or more hepatic cancers. In adults, carcinoma is associated with atrophic annular liver cirrhosis in more than 60% of cases.

Most patients with hepatoma die within 6–12 months after the primary clinical signs. In a few patients, the tumours grow slowly over a longer clinical course of one or more years.

8.3 HISTOPATHOLOGY

Both primary and metastatic malignant tumours are found in the liver. Synonyms for carcinoma of the liver include hepatoma, hepatic cell carcinoma and hepatocellular carcinoma. All are primary carcinomas of the liver which arise from the hepatic parenchymal cell. Most tumour cells bear a resemblance to cord cells, but some tumours may be extremely anaplastic.

8.4 INVESTIGATIONS

8.4.1 Medical imaging

(a) Conventional radiograph

- Hepatomegaly may be shown by plain films. If a tumour develops on the upper portion, deformities of the right hemidiaphragm may be seen.
- Arteriography may show signs of compression by surrounding tumour. Sometimes hypervascularization or other abnormal vascularization may be found.
- Portography will also show the deformities of intra-hepatic veins.

Arteriography and portography need not be carried out if other less invasive techniques are available (computed tomography and magnetic resonance imaging).

(b) Ultrasound B

Ultrasound B is the simplest non-invasive method and is the most essential technique.

(c) Radioisotopic scan

Radioisotopic gallium (^{67}Ga) and radioactive selenomethionine (^{75}Se) are often taken up by carcinomas of the liver. If radioactive colloidal gold (^{198}Au) is used, the areas involved with the tumour are colder than those not involved.

8.4.2 Laboratory findings

The erythrocyte sedimentation rate is elevated. A2 globulin and fibrinogen levels are elevated. Anaemia is present and the levels of white blood cells are elevated (around 10 000 per mm^3). Anicteric cholestasis is present. The BSP is decreased. Alkaline phosphatase levels are elevated.

8.4.3 Laparoscopy and needle biopsy

For histological documentation, a needle biopsy is necessary, but must be absolutely avoided in very vascular tumours.

8.5 STAGING AND PROGNOSIS

Tables 8.1 and 8.2 show the UICC–TNM classification system and stage groupings for liver cancer.

The prognosis for hepatoma is extremely poor. Out of 100 patients, only one has a chance of being alive five years after diagnosis. Early detection is not easy and most of the cases diagnosed are at an advanced stage. The resection rate is always lower than 10%. The five-year survival is less than 30% even when total resection of tumour is carried out.

8.6 TREATMENT – CHOICE OF MODALITY

8.6.1 Radical treatment

Selected patients with T1 tumours that are resected may have cure rates as high as 30%. Apart from this, there is no role for radical radiation therapy in this disease.

8.6.2 Palliative treatment

The development of radioimmunotherapy for hepatomas has met with apparent early success but remains an experimental modality. External beam radiation for primary hepatomas has very limited scope in relief of symptoms such as pain.

Table 8.1 UICC–TNM classification (1987)

Stage	Description
TX	Primary tumour cannot be assessed
T0	No evidence of primary tumour
T1	Solitary tumour 2 cm or less in greatest dimension without vascular invasion
T2	Solitary tumour 2 cm or less in greatest dimension with vascular invasion or multiple tumours limited to one lobe, none more than 2 cm in greatest dimension without vascular invasion or a solitary tumour more than 2 cm in greatest dimension without vascular invasion
T3	Solitary tumour more than 2 cm in greatest dimension with vascular invasion; multiple tumours limited to one lobe, none more than 2 cm in greatest dimension, with vascular invasion, or more than 2 cm in greatest dimension, with or without vascular invasion
T4	Multiple tumours in more than one lobe or tumour(s) involving a major branch of portal or hepatic vein(s)
NX	Regional lymph nodes cannot be assessed
N0	No regional lymph node metastasis
N1	Regional lymph node metastasis
MX	Presence of distant metastasis cannot be assessed
M0	No distant metastasis
M1	Distant metastasis

Table 8.2 Stage grouping (UICC, 1987)

Stage	T	N	M
I	T1	N0	M0
II	T2	N0	M0
III	T1	N1	M0
	T2	N1	M0
	T3	N0, N1	M0
IVA	T4	Any N	M0
IVB	Any T	Any N	M1

Most frequently, liver metastases are treated by systemic therapy due to the intrinsic sensitivity of the liver. Jaundice generally reflects disseminated intra-hepatic spread best treated by chemotherapy. The palliative application of radiation is primarily limited to relief of capsular pain often requiring radiation of the entire liver. Treatment regimens typically deliver 20–24 Gy in 10–12 fractions or 30 Gy in 12–15 fractions; higher total doses are not possible due to effects of radiation hepatitis. In rare circumstances where localized beams can be used, such as in portal obstruction due to adenopathy, radiation may provide benefit with less treatment-related morbidity. Regimens of 40–45 Gy can be administered with conventional fractionation. Nausea and vomiting are the most likely acute sequelae of treatment which can be prevented using pretreatment anti-emetics. However, these symptoms may often be present as a result of metastatic involvement. Nutritional and fluid supplementation are often required during radiotherapy to avoid dehydration.

8.6.3 Palliative radiotherapy

(a) Indications

Palliative radiotherapy may be used in T1, T2, M0 tumours or cases of intra-hepatic dissemination but localized to the liver with good general condition. Cirrhosis is not an absolute contra-indication, because hepatoma is always combined with cirrhosis. Of course, the response is poor in these cases. Distant metastases are rare and late, and are the only contra-indication to radiotherapy. Use in hepatoma of an inflammatory type with rapid growth is also contra-indicated.

(b) Radiotherapy techniques

Nuclear scanning computed tomography and/or magnetic resonance imaging should be used for localization when available. If laparotomy is performed, radiopaque markers should be placed *in situ*, to help the later external irradiation.

For local irradiation of T1, T2 tumours, localized target volumes may be used with opposed anterior and posterior fields. Doses to 60 Gy in 6 weeks may be attempted. For total hepatic irradiation, opposed large anterior and posterior fields are used. It is very difficult to give high doses to control hepatic malignancies. Approximately 20–25 Gy is considered the limit of tolerance.

9

Cervix

9.1 INCIDENCE AND RISK FACTORS

Cervical cancer is the second most common cancer, after breast cancer, among women worldwide. It is the most frequent cancer in women in Africa, Central America and tropical South America, China, India and other Asian countries. In North America and Europe, it is the fourth most common cancer in women. A recent increase has been reported in young women. Cervical cancer in many developing countries afflicts women with the greatest socio-economic responsibility in the community. Typically this is a 40–55 year mother of up to 15 children (average six or seven), mostly uneducated and resident in a rural area. Large differences in risk are observed within a continent or even within a given country.

The development of squamous cervical cancer is strongly linked with human sexual behaviour. Recent studies have provided some evidence for venereally transmitted aetiological agents, such as human papillomaviruses. The risk of cervical cancer is increased more than tenfold for women with six or more sexual partners or when sexual activity began before the age of 15. Male sexual promiscuity also increases the risk of cervical cancer in the female partner.

9.2 PRESENTATION AND NATURAL HISTORY

Carcinoma of the cervix is a progressive disease. It begins with intra-epithelial, preneoplastic changes which may develop over a period of ten years or more into invasive cervical cancer.

Histopathologically, pre-invasive cervical lesions usually develop through several stages of dysplasia (mid–moderate–severe) which lead to carcinoma *in situ* and finally to invasion. However, some studies have shown that up to 25% of pre-invasive lesions regress spontaneously.

The presenting symptoms of early cervical cancer are postcoital bleeding or spontaneous vaginal bleeding. In later stages, vaginal discharge, low backache, urinary and bowel symptoms appear, due to extension of the disease to the nearby structures. Further symptoms are due to paraortic lymph node enlargement and cause intensive lumbar pain and hydronephrosis. Cough due to lung metastasis and loss of appetite due to hepatic metastasis appear in very late stages.

9.3 HISTOPATHOLOGY

The majority of cervical cancers (95%) are epidermoid (most moderately differentiated, rarely anaplastic and well differentiated), 5% are adenocarcinoma, and 1% are other forms. The possibility of adenocarcinoma extending from the body of the uterus to the cervix should always be excluded by fractional curettage.

9.4 INVESTIGATIONS

The macroscopic appearance on vaginal speculum examination and visual examination is proliferative growth, ulceration or enlargement of the cervix with minimal external ulceration or growth.

Clinical examination should consist of examination of supraclavicular and other lymph node sites, examination of the abdomen, speculum examination, digital bimanual examination of the vagina, cervix, and fornices, and rectal examination. Speculum examination will help to determine the macroscopic nature of the tumour and digital examination of the rectum will determine the parametrial extension and disposition of the uterus.

Histopathological proof of invasive cancer should always be obtained by cytology, conization or simple punch biopsy.

Other essential laboratory investigations are complete blood counts and urea estimation. Low haemoglobin levels should be corrected with transfusion before treatment. A high total white blood cell count indicates uterine pyometria or cystitis, both requiring aggressive antibiotic therapy and occasionally evacuation of the uterus.

Table 9.1 Staging of carcinoma of the cervix and best reported results

UICC stage	Description	FIGO stage	Approximate five-year survival (%)
Tis	Carcinoma *in situ*	0	100
T1	Confined to cervix	1	
T1a	Micro-invasive	1a	95
T1b	Invasive	Ib	85
T2	Extension to vagina (not lower third)/parametrium (not lower third)/not pelvic wall	II	
T2a	Vagina (not lower third)	IIa	70
T2b	Parametrium/not pelvic wall	IIb	65
T3	Extension to lower third of the vagina/parametrium/pelvic wall	III	
T3a	Vagina (lower third)	IIIa	
			40
T3b	Parametrium/pelvic wall	IIIb	
T4	Extension to bladder/rectum/beyond true pelvis	IVa	5–10
M1	Distant organs	IVb	0.5

Cystoscopy may be undertaken in later stages as bladder involvement necessitates modification in therapy. Routine intravenous pyelography may occasionally indicate hydroureter even in early cases and hence may consequently help in planning combined therapy aimed at control of the disease and ureteric obstruction. Lymphography to identify paraortic nodes and a computed tomographic scan to estimate the extent of pelvic disease and paraortic nodes are not of particular value in cervical cancer.

9.5 STAGING AND PROGNOSIS

Table 9.1 indicates the relationship between survival and the stage of disease.

9.6 TREATMENT – CHOICE OF MODALITY

9.6.1 Radical treatment

Surgery and radiotherapy are equally applicable in early stage (1a) disease. The former has advantages such as preservation of sexual function and providing a chance to evaluate the status of the pelvic structures and metastatic disease. Unfortunately, in most developing countries, presentation with early stage disease is uncommon. Further, the mean age of cervical cancer patients is above 50, which makes preservation of sexual function less critical. Radiotherapy techniques in cancer of the cervix are simple and have been proven over time. They could serve as the method of choice in developing countries where the above factors are operative.

Certain pathological anatomical factors must be considered. The predominant local spread of the disease in earlier stages is to the vagina, parametrium and the lower part of the body of the uterus. In later stages, the disease spreads to the utero-sacral ligaments, bladder and rectum.

Lymph node involvement takes place regionally to the obturator, presacral and hypogastric group of lymph nodes in the pelvis and later to the paraortic lymph nodes. The incidence of involvement of these nodes in different stages is as follows: stage I 10–15%; stage II 20–30%; stage III 40–60%. In early disease, the chance of paraortic lymph node involvement is negligible.

The endometrium and vagina have very high tolerances to radiation, 300 Gy and 240 Gy respectively, whereas the bladder and rectum have relatively poor tolerance to radiation with a range of 60–75 Gy. This tolerance pattern gives the opportunity to deliver a comparatively high dose to the centre of the pelvis and necessitates reduction in dose towards the periphery in the sagittal plane.

External teletherapy helps to shrink the central tumour and provides most of the dose to the pelvic nodes. The introduction of supervoltage X-rays has simplified external teletherapy of the pelvis, with considerable reduction in morbidity.

(a) Principles of brachytherapy for carcinoma of the cervix

The pattern of spread of early cervical cancer necessitates creation of an isodose volume in the shape of a thin triangular disc. Such an isodose volume will ensure uniform irradiation of the tumour volume, sparing the bladder and rectum. This is achieved using an intracavitary source in the uterus and a pair of ovoids in the vagina. Since the lateral fall of dose with intracavitary therapy is marked, there should be certain physical reference points within the pelvis to calculate the dose received by the tumour and some of the critical structures. Point A is a point marked on the verification radiograph which is 2 cm above the lateral fornix and 2 cm lateral to the axis of the intra-uterine canal. This represents the central dose and indirectly the minimum dose received by the tumour and the paracervical tissues. From dosimetry analysis of treated cases, it was observed that dose in the paracervical triangle has a direct bearing on high-dose effects in the pelvis as well as on control of cancer in the cervix. Hence a point in the paracervical triangle is selected as the reference point. The whole treatment is programmed based on the tolerance of this point, which was found to be around 80 Gy. Point B is a point marked on the radiograph which is 3 cm more lateral than point A and represents the dose to the lymph nodes in the pelvis.

The radioactive source is placed in applicators and inserted into the uterus and vagina. These may range from simple rubber intra-uterine tubes and vaginal ovoids to sophisticated metal or polyurethane applicators available with the modern afterloading equipment.

Radium was previously used as the preloaded source in brachytherapy of cervical cancer. Because of radiation exposures and the presence of gaseous products of radium, it has now been replaced with solid radioactive sources such as ^{131}Cs and ^{60}Co. ^{131}Cs is preferred to ^{60}Co as it has a longer half-life and monochromatic energy. Further, since the gamma rays of caesium are less penetrating, radiation protection is also easier.

A technique that is widely used is manual afterloading brachytherapy in which radiation exposure to medical staff is completely avoided. Minimal exposure of the technical staff occurs with no protection to nursing staff and house officers. Remote afterloading brachytherapy uses medium- or high-dose rates and all categories of staff are fully protected from exposure to radiation. Even though remote afterloading is ideal, such equipment is extremely expensive and manual afterloading is still attractive for countries with limited resources.

Depending on the dose rate, afterloading techniques may be classified as LDR (low dose rate) when point A receives doses at a rate of 50–70 cGy per hour, MDR (medium dose rate) when point A exposure is 15–20 cGy per minute, and HDR (high dose rate) when the exposure rate to point A is > 200 cGy per minute.

Since most of the experience on tumour control and morbidity is based on radium, radiobiologically equivalent doses had to be determined before switching over from radium treatment to MDR and HDR techniques. It has been shown that a reduction of 10–12% in dose with MDR and of 35–40% with HDR will be optimal.

Apart from non-bulky stage I cervical cancer, which is treated with brachytherapy, all other stages are treated with a combination of teletherapy and brachytherapy. The approximate rates of local control achieved for different stages are: stage I 80%; stage II 65%; stage III 45–50%. External beam therapy can be administered either by a cobalt unit or a linear accelerator with a parallel pair of fields or using a box technique. If the patient has an anterior–posterior diameter of more than 18 cm, the latter will be better to minimize the lateral-edge effect.

(b) Special situations

Cervical stump cancer should be treated with a combination of external beam therapy and intracavitary application of short intrauterine tube and small ovoids. Central recurrence after radiation therapy should be treated with extrafacial hysterectomy or exenteration depending on the clinical situation. Adenocarcinoma of the cervix should be managed in the same way as squamous cancer.

9.6.2 Palliative treatment

The most common indications for palliative irradiation include pain and bleeding. Locally advanced or recurrent pelvic tumours may invade the sacral plexus and cause lymphatic, urinary or rectal obstruction. A variety of treatment schedules for external irradiation have been used to provide tumour regression sufficient to relieve symptoms.

9.7 RADIOTHERAPY TECHNIQUES

9.7.1 Radical irradiation for stage II carcinoma of the cervix

The target volume is the tumour and the iliac lymph nodes. The prescribed dose is 44 Gy to the pelvis. The technique is a four-field box technique with telecobalt.

- *Position.* Supine.
- *Localization.* Mark in the vagina; the rectum may be outlined with barium for the lateral portals.
- *Field margins* (Figures 9.1 and 9.2).
  Anterior and posterior fields (15–18 cm × 14–17 cm):

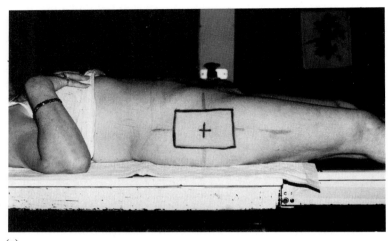

(a)

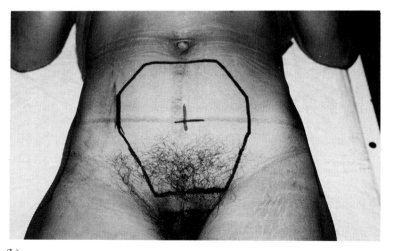

(b)

Figure 9.1 Radical irradiation. Skin marks: (a) lateral field; (b) anterior field.

upper limit: L5–S1 or L4–L5 for stage III
lower limit: the superior two-thirds of the vagina
lateral limits: 1.5 cm outside the pelvic rim

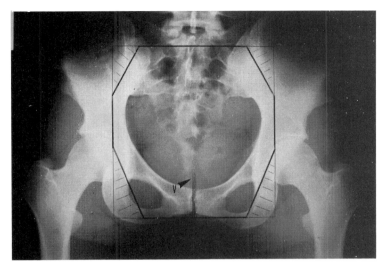

(a)

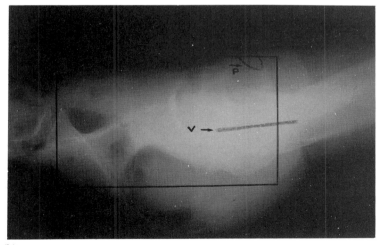

(b)

Figure 9.2 Radical irradiation. Outline of the field limits on a radiograph:
(a) anterior field; (b) lateral field. V, mark in the vagina; P, pubic bone.

Lateral fields (15–18 cm × 10–12 cm):

upper and lower limits: as above
anterior limit: mid-symphysis
posterior limit: mid-rectum

- *Beam modifications.* Blocks to shield part of the intestine and the head of femur.
- *Dose prescription* (Figure 9.3). The total dose at the axis intersection is 44 Gy in 22 fractions over 4½ weeks.
- *Special consideration.* Treatment is then completed with brachytherapy to give 70 Gy to point A and 54 Gy to the lateral pelvis but must not exceed 66 Gy to the rectum and the bladder. Depending on the total dose received on point B or the lateral

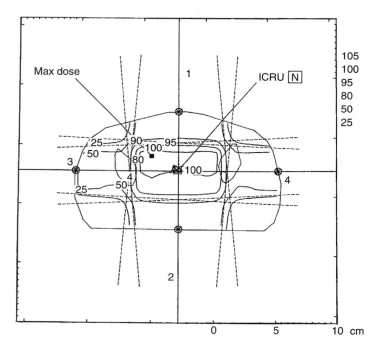

Figure 9.3 Radical irradiation. Isodose distribution for cobalt and SSD = 80 cm. [N] normalized on the 100% (ICRU) point; (■) maximum dose 102%. Loading: (1) anterior: 65 cGy/fr; (2) posterior: 65 cGy/fr; (3) right lateral: 35 cGy/fr; (4) left lateral: 35 cGy/fr.

pelvis reference point, 4–8 Gy can be added to the lateral pelvis with AP–PA fields if tumour response is modest in this area.

9.7.2 Palliative radiotherapy for stage IVb

This is used in cases of advanced tumours and old or fragile patients. The target volume will be the tumour and the surrounding tissues without intention to cover the whole pelvis. The technique involves two parallel opposed fields with telecobalt.

- *Position.* Supine.
- *Localization.* Lead mark in the vagina.
- *Field margins* (12 × 12 cm).

    upper limit: mid-sacroiliac point
    lower limit: 3 cm below the tumour
    lateral limits: 1 cm outside the pelvic rim.

- *Dose prescription.* 30 Gy in 10 fractions over 2 weeks.

9.7.3 Brachytherapy technique

This is performed 2–4 weeks after radiotherapy. The patient is under general or peridural anaesthesia.

- Careful clinical examination is performed to evaluate the response to radiotherapy. A radiopaque marker is placed in the cervix.
- Dilatation of the cervix and positioning of a gynaecological applicator (Fletcher Suit or others) after hysterometry.
- Packing of vagina.
- Afterloading of the applicator with ^{131}Cs sources in the uterine tandem and in the vaginal ovoids.
- Bladder catheter with 7 ml radiopaque dye in the balloon and marker on the anal margin and anal canal.
- *In vivo* rectal dose rate control if available.
- X-ray film control. Two orthogonal frontal and lateral films if possible.
- Calculation of dose distribution on reference points A and B. Rectal and bladder reference point. Other points if necessary.
- Duration of time is calculated to give 70 Gy to point A without exceeding the tolerance dose to rectum and bladder (66 Gy).

- Sometimes two applications can be done 1 or 2 weeks apart with half dose each.
- Antibiotics, corticoids and anticoagulant therapy may be given.

9.8 MORBIDITY

The morbidity caused by radiotherapy is mostly restricted to the structures with poor tolerance. This is due to the high dose effect because of the proximity of certain sources to some of the vital structures and the integral dose received by the pelvis. In this context, it may be worth remembering the anatomical relation of the ovoids to the rectum and the trigone of the bladder. In a retroverted uterus, the intra-uterine tube is very close to the upper rectum and rectosigmoid junction. Occasionally, a small intestinal loop within the pelvis may be close to the intra-uterine source and may be overdosed, resulting in watery diarrhoea and occasional perforation and later stricture formation. To avoid all these complications, simple precautions are required. The rectal dose can be reduced by placing a good pack between the ovoid and anterior rectum. If the bladder is continuously drained with a Foley catheter, the bladder dose can be minimized. A small intestinal loop in the pelvis may recede into the abdomen if the foot end of the bed is raised.

Radiation complications are classified as grade I when they are temporary and amenable to conventional forms of treatment. Grade II complications are more severe but will be amenable to non-surgical forms of treatment. Grade III reactions are those which require surgical correction. Grade II reactions are telangiectasia and bleeding from the bladder, rectal ulceration and long-standing tenesmus, chronic diarrhoea, sub-acute intestinal obstruction, and excessive vaginal discharge due to necrosis. The major forms of grade III reactions are contracted bladder, rectal stricture, recto-sigmoid stricture, rectosigmoid ulceration and bleeding, small gut perforation and stenosis, and rectovaginal and vesicovaginal fistulae. In any good centre, such complications should occur in less than 3% of patients. Grade I, grade II and grade III reactions together should not occur in more than 15–20% of a patient population.

Complications due to external radiation are minimal. Mild diarrhoea in the 3rd week of treatment and tenesmus are some of the complications. These can be managed by a low-residue, milk-free diet and the use of paregoric and related drugs.

Systemic diseases such as diabetes, leprosy, peripheral vascular disease and hypertension considerably increase the chance for morbidity. It may be worthwhile reducing the dose by 5–10% in such patients, especially if they are in the older age group (> 70 years old). For intractable tenesmus and rectal bleeding steroid retention enemas may help.

10

Endometrium

10.1 INCIDENCE AND RISK FACTORS

Carcinoma of the endometrium is the most common tumour in the female genital tract in the Western world, where its prevalence seems to have been increasing over the last 20 years. Most cases diagnosed are in 60–70-year-old women. Prolonged administration of exogenous hormones may be correlated with a greater risk of developing carcinoma of the endometrium. Papanicolaou smears are successful in detecting the disease in only 20–50% of cases.

10.2 PRESENTATION AND NATURAL HISTORY

The most common presenting symptom of endometrial carcinoma is abnormal uterine bleeding. Approximately 20% of patients presenting with postmenopausal bleeding in the Western world will be diagnosed as having endometrial carcinoma, but when such bleeding occurs in a woman more than 80 years old, the rate of endometrial carcinoma increases to 60%.

10.3 HISTOPATHOLOGY

Endometrial biopsy is the most accurate method of detecting endometrial carcinoma, with only a 3% false negative rate and a 3% rate of unsatisfactory specimens. Fractional dilatation and curettage is performed with tissue obtained separately from the endocervix and endometrium to make the diagnosis of endometrial carcinoma

Table 10.1 FIGO and TNM staging schemes (UICC, 1987) and five-year survival rates

FIGO stage	TNM stage	Description	Five-year survival (%)
0	Tis	Carcinoma *in situ*	100
I	T1	Carcinoma confined to the corpus uteri	90
IA	T1a	Uterine cavity $\leq$ 8 cm in length	95
IB	TIb	Uterine cavity $>$ 8 cm in length	85
		Stage 1 should be subgrouped by histology as follows: G1, highly differentiated; G2, moderately differentiated; G3, undifferentiated	
II	T2	Extension to cervix only	70
III	T3	Extension outside the uterus but confined to true pelvis	40–50
IV	T4	Extension beyond true pelvis or invading bladder or rectum	20

and to determine endocervical involvement. If involvement of the cervix is suspected biopsies should be obtained.

Adenocarcinoma is the most common tumour in the endometrium. Less commonly, the tumour may be a sarcoma which has a poorer prognosis.

10.4 INVESTIGATIONS

Clinical examination of the abdomen and the pelvis is required. Hysterography can identify the lesion inside the uterine cavity, and cystoscopy may be indicated in later stages to assess bladder involvement.

10.5 STAGING AND PROGNOSIS

Salient factors in the prognosis of endometrial carcinoma include the degree of differentiation of the tumour, the depth of myometrial invasion, the histological subtype of the tumour, and pelvic and/or paraortic lymph node involvement. Most of this information is only available after surgery, such that surgery is both diagnostic and therapeutic. Table 10.1 shows the relationship between survival and the stage of disease.

10.6 TREATMENT – CHOICE OF MODALITY

10.6.1 Radical treatment

The mainstay of treatment of endometrial carcinoma is total hysterectomy which should be undertaken whenever possible.

(a) Stage IA

Patients may be subdivided into two groups.

1. Those with well and moderately differentiated adenocarcinoma who are treated with a wide-cuff hysterectomy. If the myometrial involvement is less than one half of the wall thickness, no further therapy with irradiation is required. These patients have a less than 5% chance of vaginal recurrences after hysterectomy and vigilance in follow-up should identify such recurrences early enough for effective treatment. Alternatively post-operative intravaginal brachytherapy for all patients may reduce the 5% vaginal recurrence to negligible levels but at a cost of unnecessary radiation side-effects to a majority of the patients.
2. Patients with poorly differentiated tumours are infrequent in stage IA and should be treated with post-operative irradiation as in stage IB and stage II.

(b) Stage IB and stage II

Several therapy options for adjuvant radiotherapy have been suggested for this category of patients. One option is external beam irradiation to the pelvis and brachytherapy to the vagina.

(c) Stage III

These patients are considered technically inoperable so that radiotherapy alone forms their best treatment option. Similar radiotherapy field arrangements are used as for stages IB and II. Treatment consists of whole-pelvis external irradiation with additional irradiation delivered to the parametria. This may be combined with intracavitary brachytherapy.

10.6.2 Palliative treatment

Patients with stage IV disease are essentially palliative cases. External irradiation is used to provide tumour regression and relieve symptoms such pain and bleeding.

10.7 RADIOTHERAPY TECHNIQUES – POST-OPERATIVE IRRADIATION

This is performed 4–6 weeks after total hysterectomy and bilateral adnexectomy. The target volume is the pelvis and vagina. The prescribed dose is 46 Gy to this volume. The technique is a four-field box technique with telecobalt.

- *Position.* Supine.
- *Localization.* Mark in the vagina; the rectum may be outlined with barium for the lateral fields.
- *Field margins.*
  Anterior and posterior fields (15–18 cm × 14–17 cm):

  > upper limit: L5–S1
  > lower limit: superior two-thirds of the vagina
  > lateral limits: 1 cm outside the pelvic rim

  Lateral fields (15–18 cm × 10–12 cm):

  > upper and lower limits: as above
  > anterior limit: mid-pubic bone
  > posterior limit: mid-rectum

- *Beam modifications.* Blocks to shield part of the intestine and head of femur.
- *Dose prescription.* The total dose at the axis intersection is 46 Gy in 23 frs over $4\frac{1}{2}$ weeks.
- *Special consideration.* After a 2-week rest, the dose is completed with brachytherapy of the vagina: 20 Gy at low dose rate or two sequences of 7 Gy at the surface of the vagina 1 week apart using high dose rate.

11

Ovary

11.1 INCIDENCE AND RISK FACTORS

Ovarian cancers originate from diverse cell types. Overall incidence rates vary from 4 to 30 per 100 000 women. The rates in Africa and Asia appear to be lower than in the West. Each tumour type probably has differing aetiological factors which remain generally unknown.

11.2 PRESENTATION AND NATURAL HISTORY

The diagnosis of ovarian cancer should be suspected when any woman complains of abdominal distention, abdominal pain, constipation, urinary obstruction and backache. A gynaecological examination should invariably be undertaken. An ultrasound examination of the pelvis and abdomen will give additional information on gynaecological pathology. Exploration of the abdomen should be undertaken under the following conditions as the possibility of an adnexal mass being malignant is high: mass greater than 8 cm, increase in size or persistence through two or three menstrual cycles, solid and irregular mass, fixed or bilateral mass, and pain or ascites.

Determination of the histological nature of the disease and staging are possible only through exploratory laparotomy. In patients with poor general health and advanced disease, where a laparotomy is impossible, diagnosis can justifiably be made through cytological examination of the ascitic fluid, fine-needle aspiration cytology, percutaneous true-cut biopsy and other simple methods of diagnosis. Laparoscopy and computed tomographic scans should not be relied on solely for staging ovarian tumours as the information provided lacks specificity and sensitivity.

Because of the insidious onset of ovarian cancer, clinical symptoms in early stages are absent or minimal. Later, 50–75% of the patients will have abdominal, urinary or gynaecological symptoms singly or in combination. A high level of clinical suspicion helps to diagnose these cases. The clinical signs may be abdominal or pelvic tumours or tumours extending from the pelvis to the abdomen with or without ascites. Usually there is rapid weight loss, anaemia, occasionally unexplained fever, and in later stages evidence of cachexia.

11.3 HISTOPATHOLOGY

The World Health Organization classification of malignant ovarian tumours is extensive and complicated.

A simple listing in order of decreasing frequency is:

- epithelial tumours

    serous
    mucinous
    endometrioid

- mesodermal tumours

    stromal sarcomas
    Mullerian mixed tumours
    Brenner tumours

- granulosa-cell tumours
- androblastomas
- germ-cell tumours

    dysgerminoma
    choriocarcinoma

- teratomas

Epithelial tumours are either benign, malignant or of low malignant potential. The latter tumours have a slow progression and long natural history. Almost all are curable with surgical treatment unless the disease is advanced.

Tumour grade has an important prognostic significance in epithelial neoplasms. Grade I serous, mucinous and endometrial tumours carry a more favourable outlook than moderately differentiated, poorly differentiated and unclassified serous tumours.

Among the stromal tumours which constitute 10% of all ovarian cancer, granulosa-cell tumours are the most common. The clinical progression of these tumours varies from indolent to highly malignant.

Germ-cell tumours fall into three major groups: dysgerminomas, which are similar to testicular seminomas in pathological appearance, predominant lymphatic spread and high radiosensitivity; endodermal sinus tumours which are highly malignant; and rapidly progressive ovarian neoplasms with characteristic Schiller–Dual bodies and presence of tumour markers such as human chronic genadotrophin and alpha-fetoprotein. These are derived from the extra-embryonal tissues. Embryonic carcinoma is another variety of germ-cell tumour which is extremely rare and associated with the presence of tumour markers such as human chorionic gonadotrophin and alpha-fetoprotein. Endodermal sinus tumours are extremely sensitive to current chemotherapy methods and are highly curable.

11.4 INVESTIGATIONS

Investigations required include:

- physical examination, blood counts, renal function tests;
- pelvic examination;
- ultrasound scan of the abdomen;
- cytology of the ascitic fluid if present;
- exploratory laparotomy.

11.5 STAGING AND PROGNOSIS

Table 11.1 shows the FIGO classification system for ovarian carcinoma. Staging is always surgical and is based on an exploratory laparotomy unless this cannot be undertaken due to medical problems and poor general health. The five-year survival is shown in Table 11.2.

Table 11.1 FIGO stage grouping for carcinoma of the ovary (UICC, 1987)

Stage	Description
I	Growth limited to the ovaries.
IA	Growth limited to one ovary; no ascites. No tumour on the external surface, capsule intact.
IB	Growth limited to both ovaries; no ascites. No tumour on the external surfaces; capsules intact.
IC*	Tumour is either stage IA or IB but is on the surface of one or both ovaries, or with capsule(s) ruptured, or with ascites present containing malignant cells, or with positive peritoneal washings.
II	Growth involving one or both ovaries with pelvic extension.
IIA	Growth involving one or both ovaries with pelvic extension.
IIB	Extension and/or metastases to the uterus and/or tubes
IIC	Tumour is either stage IIA or IIB but is on the surface of one or both ovaries, or with capsule(s) ruptured, or with positive peritoneal washings.
III	Tumour involving one or both ovaries with peritoneal implants outside the pelvis and/or positive retroperitoneal or inguinal nodes. Superficial liver metastases equal stage III. Tumour is limited to the true pelvis but with histologically verified malignant extension to small bowel or omentum.
IIIA	Tumour grossly limited to the true pelvis with negative nodes but with histologically confirmed microscopic seeding of abdominal peritoneal surfaces.
IIIB	Tumour of one or both ovaries with histologically confirmed implants of abdominal peritoneal surfaces, not exceeding 2 cm in diameter. Nodes negative.
IIIC*	Abdominal implants greater than 2 cm in diameter and/or positive retroperitoneal or inguinal nodes.
IV	Growth involving one or both ovaries with distant metastasis. If pleural effusion is present, there must be positive cytological test results to allot a case to stage IV. Parenchymal liver metastasis equals stage IV.

*To determine the prognosis for stages IC or IIC, it is of value to know whether rupture of the capsule was spontaneous or caused by the surgeon, and whether the source of malignant cells detected was peritoneal washings or ascites.

11.6 TREATMENT – CHOICE OF MODALITY

11.6.1 Radical treatment

Treatment will depend on the stage and clinical presentation. Stage I epithelial tumours require only surgical treatment in almost all

Table 11.2 Relationship between stage and survival

Stage	Five-year survival (%)
I	75
II	60
III	20
IV	0

situations. The surgery should consist of a panhysterectomy and sampling of all tissues likely to be involved in the disease process except in certain special situations. Stage II tumours require a panhysterectomy and whole-abdominal radiation (now rarely employed) with pelvic boost to be undertaken if the size of the residual nodules is < 2 cm. If > 2 cm, chemotherapy with the single agent *cis*-platin is preferable.

For stage III tumours, a panhysterectomy or maximum possible debulking followed by administration of chemotherapy with a combination of *cis*-platin and drugs such as cyclophosphamide, fluorouracil or adriamycin is the treatment of choice. The number of courses required to achieve a complete remission varies from four to six. Residual tumour at the end of chemotherapy is either resected or irradiated with localized fields of up to 30 Gy in 10 fractions. In the alternative situation when only biopsy is done, chemotherapy is employed and residual disease (if resectable) is resected at the end of the four to six courses of chemotherapy. If surgical resection is not feasible, radiotherapy can be used to consolidate the gains of chemotherapy.

(a) Dysgerminoma

As this tumour occurs in young women and the probability of cure is high (80–90%), these women require special consideration with regard to therapy. As 90% of these tumours are unilateral, oophorectomy followed by chemotherapy using a combination of *cis*-platin and etoposide is justifiable in young patients who want to complete their families. As no reliable tumour marker is available for this tumour, it is necessary to monitor these patients clinically and ultrasonically for recurrence to facilitate early intervention. All other early-stage patients are preferably treated with post-operative radiation therapy to the abdomen after panhysterectomy as the lymph node metastases are extremely radiosensitive. In stage III disease, where the chance of haematogenous metastasis is high, the preferred line of treatment is again chemotherapy.

(b) Endodermal sinus tumour

Endodermal sinus tumours are rarely surgically excisable as they are widely disseminated within the abdominal cavity even at the time of initial presentation. Chemotherapy for 4–6 months using a combination of two or three drugs comprising *cis*-platin, etoposide, vinblastine or bleomycin will achieve complete remission in 70% of cases. Radiotherapy does not have any role in the management of this condition.

(c) Granulosa-cell tumour

Recurrent granulosa-cell tumours should always be excised if they are operable. Chemotherapy in inoperable recurrences, especially using adriamycin, has been found to be useful.

11.6.2 Palliative treatment

The present role for radiotherapy is generally limited to the palliation of recurrent cancers that are not chemotherapy responsive. The previously advocated techniques of whole-abdominal radiation therapy have been abandoned. Intracavitary radioisotope therapy has few advocates. Radiotherapy of a recurrent pelvic tumour that is producing pain or lower extremity lymphoedema can be offered with moderate success.

11.7 RADIOTHERAPY TECHNIQUES

11.7.1 Radical post-operative radiotherapy

This is performed 4–6 weeks after radical surgery in cases of high-risk recurrence in the abdominal cavity but with no residual nodules > 2 cm in diameter (stage II). The target volume will depend on the clinical delineation of the recurrence. It include the whole abdomen with a boost to pelvis and lumbo-aortic nodes. The prescribed dose is about 20 Gy on the abdomen, 30 Gy on the lumbo-aortic nodes and 45 Gy on the pelvis. The technique involves two parallel AP–PA fields with telecobalt.

- *Position.* Supine for the anterior field and prone for the posterior one.
- *Field margins.*
  Anterior and posterior abdominal fields (40 × 25 cm):

  upper limit: 1 cm above the right diaphragm
  lower limit: lower end of the foramen
  external limits: border of the abdominal cavity

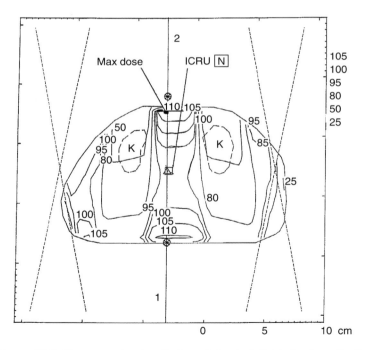

Figure 11.1 Post-operative irradiation, abdominal field. Isodose distribution for cobalt and SSD = 80 cm. $\boxed{N}$ normalized on the 100% (ICRU) point; (■) maximum dose 114%. Loading: (1) anterior: 80 cGy/fr; (2) posterior: 80 cGy/fr. K, kidney.

Anterior and posterior pelvic fields (15–18 × 25 cm):

upper limit: above the iliac bones
lower and external limits: as above

- *Beam modifications.* Blocks on AP–PA fields to spare the femoral heads and the left pulmonary basis, and on the posterior field to limit the dose to the kidney to 15 Gy.
- *Dose prescription* (Figures 11.1, 11.2 and 11.3). The total dose at the axis intersection is 22 Gy in 14 fractions over 3 weeks to the abdomen. The total dose is 31 Gy in 19 fractions over 4 weeks on the lumbo-aortic nodes, and 45 Gy in 26 fractions over 5 weeks on the pelvis.
- *Special consideration.* Whenever possible, irradiation should be given with X-ray beams of 10 to 20 MV.

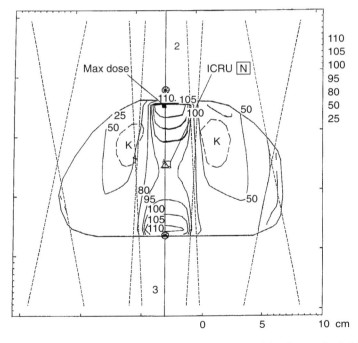

Figure 11.2 Post-operative irradiation, abdominal and lumbo-aortic fields. Isodose distribution for cobalt and SSD = 80 cm. [N] normalized on the 100% (ICRU) point; (■) maximum dose 115%. Loading: (1) anterior: 80 cGy/fr; (2) posterior: 80 cGy/fr; (3) reduced anterior: 90 cGy/fr; (4) reduced posterior: 90 cGy/fr. K, kidney.

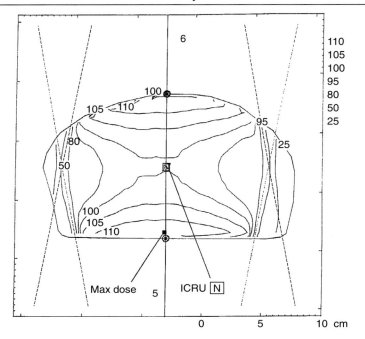

Figure 11.3 Post-operative irradiation, abdominal and pelvic fields. Isodose distribution for cobalt and SSD = 80 cm. $\boxed{N}$ normalized on the 100% point; (■) maximum dose 115%. Loading: (1) anterior: 80 cGy/fr; (2) posterior: 80 cGy/fr; (3) reduced anterior: 100 cGy/fr; (4) reduced posterior: 100 cGy/fr. K, kidney.

11.8 MORBIDITY

The palliative treatment should be designed to minimize any morbidity. The structures at risk include large and small bowel and bladder.

12

Choriocarcinoma

Gestational trophoblastic disease (GTD) is a generic term for a group of benign and malignant neoplasms derived from the trophoblast of the human placenta. Though histologically diverse, the various forms of GTD share several common features such as derivation from the human placenta, paternal genome contribution, and secretion of human chorionic gonadotrophin (hCG).

12.1 CLINICAL CLASSIFICATION

Trophoblastic disease is clinically classified as benign or malignant, and the malignant category is further subdivided into metastatic and non-metastatic. Tumours with a pathological diagnosis of choriocarcinoma or invasive mole always behave as malignant lesions and require therapy, whereas hydatidiform moles can be benign (80%) or malignant (20%) based on their clinical course.

Patients often present with vaginal haemorrhage and spontaneous abortion of atypical hydropic vesicles. Benign theca-lutin cysts of the ovary are detected in approximately 20% of patients with complete moles.

The clinical diagnosis of molar gestation is confirmed by the characteristic ultrasonographic findings of mixed echogenic foci described as the 'snowstorm' pattern. Serum ß-hCG levels are markedly elevated in patients with hydatidiform mole, although a single serum hCG measurement is not a reliable diagnostic test to establish the diagnosis of hydatidiform mole.

Once the diagnosis has been made, the following investigations are recommended prior to uterine evacuations:

- complete physical and pelvic examinations;
- complete blood count;
- blood chemistries including kidney, liver and thyroid function tests;
- baseline serum hCG level;
- chest radiograph;
- pelvic ultrasonography.

12.2 INCIDENCE AND RISK FACTORS

Hydatidiform mole occurs in approximately 0.2–2 per 1000 pregnancies in India. Choriocarcinoma is far less common than hydatidiform mole, its incidence being 0.2–1 per 10 000 pregnancies. Fifty seven per cent of cases of choriocarcinoma occur after hydatidiform mole, 26% after normal pregnancy and 17% following abortion.

Women above the age of 40 years have a fivefold higher risk of trophoblastic disease when compared to mothers aged 21–35 years. There is slightly increased risk for women less than 20 years old. There is an increased risk of GTD in women with early spontaneous abortion. No other factors such as race, socio-economic status and nutrition are significant risk factors by themselves.

12.2.1 Cytogenetics

Cytogenetically hydatidiform mole can be divided into two groups, complete or partial moles. Complete moles are potentially malignant and carry a diploid component of exclusively paternal chromosomes with a 46 XX karyotype. Partial moles have a triploid (69) karyotype and carry no risk of malignancy.

12.3 HISTOPATHOLOGY

Based on the histopathological appearance, GTD is classified into hydatidiform mole, invasive mole or choriocarcinoma.

The pathological characteristics of the classic or complete hydatidiform mole are the following (the last two being the most important):

- marked oedema and enlargement of the villi;
- disappearance of the villous blood vessels;

- proliferation of the lining trophoblast of the villi;
- absence of fetal tissue.

Partial moles have identifiable fetal tissues and edematous villi, with no trophoblastic proliferation.

Invasive mole is characterized by moles with abnormal penetrativeness and extensive local invasion along with excessive trophoblastic proliferation with a well-preserved villous pattern. In choriocarcinoma, the tumour appears as a dark, haemorrhagic mass with ulceration. Microscopically, it is characterized by disorderly proliferation of trophoblastic tissue invading into the muscle with destruction and coagulation necrosis.

It is not uncommon to find complete disparity between the histological appearance and the clinical course of the disease.

12.4 MANAGEMENT

12.4.1 Hydatidiform mole

Once the diagnosis of hydatidiform mole has been made, evacuation of the uterus, preferably by suction curettage, is required, and hCG titres return to undetectable levels within 8–12 weeks. The routine use of prophylatic chemotherapy at the time of initial evacuation of a hydatidiform mole is not recommended. However, careful follow-up is indicated after evacuation because 15% of patients have persistent or invasive moles and 3–5% develop choriocarcinoma. Recommendations for follow-up include pelvic examination, weekly monitoring of the serum ß-hCG level until normal for successive weeks, then monthly monitoring for one year. Pregnancy should be avoided during the first year of follow-up.

12.4.2 Malignant trophoblastic diseases

After pretreatment evaluation, the patient is classified according to Figure 12.1. FIGO has adopted a staging system for malignant GTD, which correlates little with survival. Clinical classification of GTD is as non-metastatic or metastatic.

Low-risk patients are those without any of the following high-risk factors:

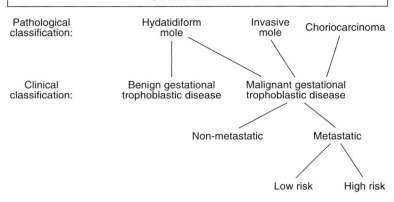

Figure 12.1 Classification scheme for gestational trophoblastic disease.

Table 12.1 Chemotherapy for malignant GTD

GTD status	Primary chemotherapy	Salvage
Non-metastatic	Single agent (MTS/FA)	Single agent (Act-D) or combination chemotherapy
Low-risk metastatic	Single agent (MTS/FA)	Single agent (Act-D) or combination chemotherapy
High-risk metastatic	Combination chemotherapy	Other combination chemotherapy

MTS, methotrexate; FA, folinic acid; Act-D, dactinomycin-D

- serum ß-hCG level higher than 40 000 mIU/ml
- disease of more than 4 months' duration
- brain and/or liver metastasis
- previous term pregnancy.

The World Health Organization has formalized an elaborate scoring system to define the risk groups that correlate well with survival after chemotherapy. Since the development of the anti-metabolite methotrexate in 1950s, chemotherapy (Table 12.1) has become the cornerstone in the treatment of malignant GTD. Indications for chemotherapy are:

- histological diagnosis of choriocarcinoma
- evidence of metastatic disease
- a plateaued or rising serum ß-hCG level after evacuation of a hydatidiform mole
- an elevated ß-hCG level after attainment of a normal serum level.

Drugs active against malignant GTD include methotrexate, dactinomycin, alkylating agents, vinca alkaloids, *cis*-platin, 5-fluorouracil and VP-16.

(a) Non-metastatic GTD

Single-agent chemotherapy with methotrexate or dactinomycin is the treatment of choice for non-metastatic GTD. Eighty to ninety-five per cent of patients can be cured with the initial agent and the rest can be salvaged by second-line therapy. In an effort to increase the dose of methotrexate and reduce toxicity, folinic acid rescue is used with methotrexate. Methotrexate (1 mg/kg intramuscularly) is administered on days 1, 3, 5 and 7, and folinic acid (0.1 mg/kg) is given on days 2, 4, 6 and 8. The courses are repeated as soon as the patient recovers from the toxicity of the primary chemotherapy.

(b) Metastatic GTD

For low-risk GTD, the same line of treatment is followed as for non-metastatic GTD. The most common chemotherapy for high-risk GTD is a combination of methotrexate, dactinomycin and chlorambucil or cyclophosphamide (MAC). Other examples of currently used combinations include the modified Bagshawe regime, hydroxyurea/methotrexate/vincristine/cyclophosphamide/dactinomycin/adriamycin and EMA/CO or a combination of VP-16, methotrexate, dactinomycin, cyclophosphamide and vincristine.

In all chemotherapy regimens, the cycle of chemotherapy is repeated as soon as the patient recovers from the toxicity of the prior chemotherapy. Chemotherapy is continued until serum ß-hCG levels attain the normal value. Thereafter, one to three more cycles of chemotherapy are given. With the recent availability of sensitive ß-hCG assay techniques, these extra courses of therapy may not be necessary in the low-risk group. For the high-risk group, two to six additional cycles of chemotherapy are advocated.

(c) Surgery

Hysterectomy is important in the management of GTD. Indications for surgery include:

- drug resistance or toxicity, with disease confined to the uterus;
- complications such as vaginal haemorrhage, uterine perforation and infection;
- older multiparous patients with localized disease.

(d) Radiation therapy

Patients with metastases to the brain or liver may develop haemorrhage, as a result of necrosis from chemotherapy. In such cases, a 20 Gy dose of external radiation to the tumour is given in 10–14 fractions, in conjunction with combination chemotherapy.

(e) Central nervous system disease

Levels of cerebrospinal fluid hCG should be monitored in the following situations:

- serum ß-hCG > 40 000 mIU/ml;
- presence of pulmonary metastasis;
- clinical suspicion of central nervous system disease.

The results are considered to be significant if the ratio of cerebrospinal fluid hCG to serum hCG is more than 1:60.

(f) Follow-up

All cases are followed up with monthly hCG assays for at least one year, even after achievement of normal hCG levels. After one year, a high-risk GTD patient should be seen twice yearly for five years and then annually. Levels of ß-hCG are checked at each visit. Patients are counselled to avoid pregnancy throughout the first year of hCG surveillance.

(g) Results

Using chemotherapy, 100% of patients with non-metastatic disease and 70% or more of high-risk patients can be cured. It is important that all patients be accurately evaluated and treated appropriately and aggressively from the outset.

13

Prostate

13.1 INCIDENCE AND RISK FACTORS

Carcinoma of the prostate is the second commonest cancer and third leading cause of cancer death in men in most developed countries. The highest world incidence rate is in black males in the San Francisco Bay area and the lowest is in Osaka, Japan (77 and 2.7 per 100 000 respectively). Rates for African blacks are lower than for American blacks. The following are age-adjusted rates per 100 000: Nigerians 10.2, South Africans 9.4, Ugandans 4.4.

Carcinoma of the prostate is rare below the age of 40 but the incidence increases exponentially with age thereafter. There is some association with higher socio-economic status and a slight familial tendency. Some studies have found higher rates in married versus single men, and also higher rates in sexually active and fertile men, but in each case other studies have given conflicting results. Heavy drinkers and those with liver cirrhosis are less likely to develop the disease, probably because a cirrhotic liver is unable metabolize oestrogens.

Environmental factors are suggested by a higher incidence of prostate cancer in succeeding generations of migrants from a low- to a high-incidence area, e.g. Japanese emigrating to North America. Dietary studies of prostate cancer mortality have shown a positive correlation with intake of meat, fats, milk and sugar but a negative correlation with consumption of cereals, pulses and rice.

13.2 PRESENTATION AND NATURAL HISTORY

Early prostate cancer is usually asymptomatic. In more advanced disease, there may be obliteration of the median sulcus or the tumour may spread laterally to the pelvic walls or superiorly to the seminal vesicles.

Since over 75% of the tumours arise in the posterior or peripheral part of the gland, symptoms of an enlarged prostate (hesitancy or urgency of micturition, a narrow stream and nocturia) are late events. Ten per cent of these tumours are discovered during prostatectomy for apparently benign prostatic hypertrophy. Perineal pain may occur either early or late in the disease. Haematuria is uncommon and relates to infection or erosion of the gland. Many patients present with bone pain or stiffness from secondary deposits, especially in the back or pelvis.

Carcinoma of the prostate generally runs an indolent course although this is variable. Clinically the tumour behaves in the same way in all races and all age groups after standardizing for stage, grade and treatment. Histological grade has a major influence on survival (60% five-year survival for well-differentiated tumours versus 10% for poorly differentiated tumours). A raised acid phosphatase level at diagnosis is associated with a poor prognosis.

13.3 HISTOPATHOLOGY

Most carcinomas of the prostate gland arise from the acinar epithelium of the peripheral zone and are adenocarcinomas. Less commonly, transitional-cell carcinomas are seen, which arise from the ductal epithelium.

Bladder tumours may spread directly into the prostate. Most prostatic carcinomas are well differentiated and mitoses are uncommon except in anaplastic tumours. Various histoprognostic scores exist. Gleason has proposed a score based on the glandular differentiation of the tumour: 2–4 indicate well differentiated, 7–10 indicate poorly differentiated.

The cytoplasm of prostatic cancer cells may contain large amounts of acid phosphatase.

13.4 INVESTIGATIONS

Once the diagnosis of prostate cancer is suspected, levels of prostate-specific antigen and acid phosphatases should be determined and rectal examination performed for staging. The examiner should note the size and consistency of the gland, any induration or nodularity, whether the lateral sulcus is involved and any spread to pelvic wall or superiorly. The finding of a firm area above the prostate suggests that the seminal vesicles are invaded by tumour.

Histological confirmation is essential for diagnosis and this is normally by needle biopsy, either transrectal or transperineal. Using the transrectal route, it is easier to place the needle accurately into the suspicious area, but the incidence of infection is higher than with the transperineal route. Ultrasonically guided needle biopsies are now prevalent.

Chest radiograph and isotope bone scans are essential and may show metastatic disease. Abnormal areas on the scan should be investigated further by radiography. An intravenous urogram may show prostatic or bladder irregularity or obstructive uropathy.

In patients who are candidates for radical surgery or radical radiotherapy, an assessment of the primary plus nodal disease is essential. Bipedal lymphangiography is the best single investigation for this purpose but has a high false-negative rate.

Computed tomographic scans are of little value unless the nodes are larger than 2 cm. Ultrasound, especially intrarectal, is being increasingly used and is highly informative in experienced hands.

13.5 STAGING AND PROGNOSIS

The most commonly used classifications are the TNM system of the UICC and the Whitmore–Jewett system (Table 13.1). The TNM system has the advantage of separating out assessment of the primary tumour from that of the nodes and metastatic disease. Its disadvantage lies in grouping together all T0 tumours although the well-differentiated and the poorly differentiated have very different prognoses. Pathological classification is denoted by the prefix p, e.g. pT, pN and pM. There is considerable discrepancy between clinical and pathological staging – one study found that in 262 tumours clinically classified as T1 or T2, 52.3% were upstaged to pT3, while of 152 clinical T3 tumours 15.1% were downstaged to pT2.

There is a clear correlation between staging and prognosis in this disease. Clinical stages T1, T2, T3 and T4 have five-year survival rates of 95, 76, 69 and 13% respectively. Other studies have shown a very significant difference in survival between those patients with disease limited to the prostate and those with extracapsular disease

Table 13.1 Classification of prostate cancer

Whitmore–Jewett staging system		UICC (1987) TNM staging system	
Stage	Description	Stage	Description
A1	Microscopic focus of well-differentiated adenocarcinoma in up to three foci of transurethral specimens or enucleation; clinically not apparent on rectal examination	T0 T1 (a) (b) T2	No tumour palpable Tumour is incidental finding < 3 microscopic foci > 3 microscopic foci Palpable tumour confined to gland
A2	Tumour not well differentiated or present in more than three areas	(a) (b)	< 1.5 cm with normal tissue around > 1.5 cm or in more than one lobe
B1	Asymptomatic palpable nodule < 1.5 cm; normal surrounding prostate; no capsular extension; normal acid phosphatase levels	T3	Invasion of prostatic apex, capsule, bladder neck or seminal vesicle but not fixed
B2	Diffuse involvement of gland; no capsular extension; normal acid phosphatase levels	T4	Tumour fixed or invading other adjacent structures
C	Extensive local tumour with penetration through the capsule, contiguous spread; may involve seminal vesicles, bladder neck, lateral side wall of pelvis; acid phosphatase levels may be elevated; normal bone scan	N0–N3 M1	As bladder cancer (Table 14.1) Distant metastases
D1	Metastases to pelvic lymph nodes below aortic bifurcation; acid phosphatase levels may be elevated		
D2	Bone or lymph node metastases above aortic bifurcation or other soft tissue metastases		

(44% versus 28%, respectively). Many studies have reported survival rates of 75–80% at five years, 60% at ten years and 35–40% at 15 years following radical prostatectomy. After radical radiotherapy, with tumour localized to the prostate, disease-free survival is about 75% at five years and 60% at ten years. In patients with extracapsular extension the results are 50% and 30% respectively.

13.6 TREATMENT – CHOICE OF MODALITY

13.6.1 Radical treatment

There is still controversy regarding the treatment of patients with localized disease, with some saying that localized treatment makes no impact in such an indolent disease occurring in an elderly population.

The two approaches are radical prostatectomy and radical radiotherapy. The former involves *en bloc* resection of the prostate, prostatic urethra and seminal vesicles with part of the surrounding connective tissue. Only patients with disease confined to the prostate and without node spread are suitable for radical surgery. Thus, radical radiotherapy is more widely applicable. Although either treatment must be considered with great care in these patients, many of whom are 65 years old, radical surgery demands a higher degree of fitness than the radiotherapeutic approach – a factor which may distort survival statistics unless clinical trials are strictly randomized.

13.6.2 Palliative treatment

In patients with advanced disease there are multiple treatment options and the choice in a particular patient will depend on the precise symptoms.

Both orchidectomy and oestrogen therapy are valuable as palliation especially in patients with bone metastases. Patients often dislike orchidectomy. Unfortunately oestrogen therapy is associated with painful gynaecomastia and a high incidence of cardiovascular side-effects, especially in patients with a previous cardiac history. Low-dose oestrogen is now used, e.g. 0.2–1 mg daily of diethylstilbestrol which is as good in terms of survival as 5 mg daily. Gynaecomastia can be prevented by prior irradiation of the nipples (section 13.7.4). The use of leuprolide, by depot intramuscular injection, 7.5 mg monthly plus flutamide, 750 mg daily by mouth has largely replaced oestrogen therapy. There is no difference in survival in advanced prostate cancer patients if hormone treatment is delayed until symptoms develop. For instance, in a patient with asymptomatic bone metastases, hormone treatment can be withheld until symptoms demand, so reducing side-effects.

Since the majority of metastases are bony and thus painful, radiotherapy has an important part to play in palliation. Single or multiple-fraction therapy doses can be given to painful tumour sites or to prevent fracture, but single-fraction half-body radiation is also increasingly used. Radiotherapy may be used for localized bone pain. For more generalized bone pain, half-body radiation is appropriate. Where urinary symptoms predominate, pelvic radiation may be indicated, even in patients with metastatic disease. Many of these patients develop pathological fractures, and, if these are detected early, and the patient is surgically immobilized and given postoperative radiotherapy, these patients may remain independent with a useful quality of life for a reasonable length of time.

Morphine is an important part of the management of the terminal phases of this disease. It should be given regularly, preferably in tablet form, with a regular laxative.

13.7 RADIOTHERAPY TECHNIQUES

13.7.1 Radical irradiation of the prostate

This is proposed for true T1 tumours (A2). In patients in whom a transurethral resection has been performed, radiation treatment should be delayed for about four weeks, otherwise the incidence of incontinence and urethral strictures is high. Concomitant hormone treatment has not been shown to improve survival and is not recommended. A variety of radiation techniques can be used. The use of anterior and posterior fields alone is not satisfactory. The target volume is the prostate and seminal vesicles. The prescribed dose is 64 Gy. The recommended technique is a four-field box technique with telecobalt.

- *Position.* Supine with a fully distended bladder.
- *Localization.* Marks on anal margin, small Foley catheter with dye in urethra and bladder, and barium in the rectum.
- *Field margins.*
  The field sizes are usually 8–10 cm × 8–10 cm:

  upper limit: 2 cm above the prostate
  lower limit: lower border of the ischial tuberosities
  anterior limit: between the anterior and middle third of the pubic bone

posterior limit: mid-rectum
lateral limits: 2 cm lateral to the prostate

- *Dose prescription* (Figure 13.1).
  The total dose is 64 Gy in 32 fractions over $6\frac{1}{2}$ weeks.

13.7.2 Radical irradiation of the prostate and pelvis

This is recommended for more advanced tumours such as T3 treated with curative intent and with a risk of lymph node involvement which cannot be neglected. The target volume covers the pelvic lymph nodes draining the prostate and seminal vesicles as in section 13.7.1. The prescribed dose is 44 Gy to the pelvis and 68 Gy to the prostate. The technique is a four-field box technique with shrinking fields using telecobalt.

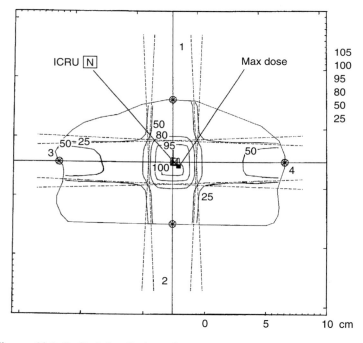

Figure 13.1 Radical irradiation of the prostate. Isodose distribution for cobalt and SSD = 80 cm. [N] normalized on the 100% (ICRU) point; (■) maximum dose 101%. Loading: (1) anterior: 65 cGy/fr; (2) posterior: 65 cGy/fr; (3) right lateral: 35 cGy/fr; (4) left lateral: 35 cGy/fr.

- *Position.* Supine with a fully distended bladder.
- *Localization.* Marks on anal margin, small Foley catheter with dye in urethra and bladder; the rectum may be outlined with barium for the lateral portals.
- *Field margins* (Figures 13.2 and 13.3).

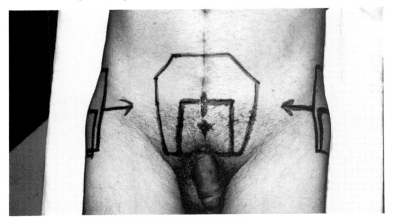

(a)

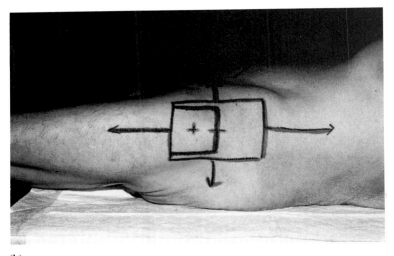

(b)

Figure 13.2 Radical irradiation of the prostate and pelvis. Skin marks: (a) anterior field; (b) lateral field.

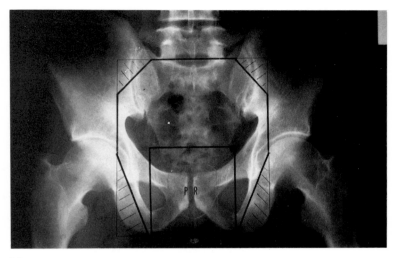

(a)

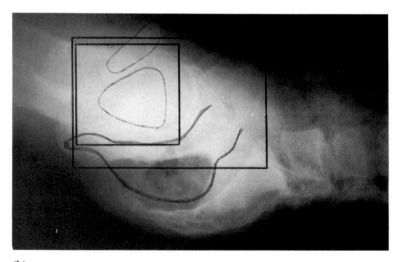

(b)

Figure 13.3 Radical irradiation of the prostate and pelvis. Outline of the field limits on a radiograph: (a) anterior field; (b) lateral field. P, pubic bone; PR, prostate; A, anal margin.

Pelvis:

> upper limit: L5–S1
> lateral limit: 1 cm outside the pelvic rim
> lower limit: lower border of the ischial tuberosities to cover the whole prostate with a safety margin of 2 cm below the apex
> anterior limit: between the anterior and middle third of the pubic bone
> posterior limit: mid-rectum

Prostate: same as section 13.7.1

- *Beam modification.* For the pelvic field, blocks are positioned to protect part of the small bowel and the head of the femur.
- *Dose prescription* (Figure 13.4). The dose to the pelvis is 44 Gy in 22 fractions over $4\frac{1}{2}$ weeks, then 24 Gy to the prostate in 12 fractions over $2\frac{1}{2}$ weeks.

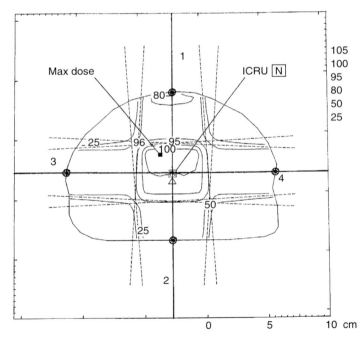

Figure 13.4 Radical irradiation of the pelvis. Isodose distribution for cobalt and SSD = 80 cm. [N] normalized on the 100% (ICRU) point; (■) maximum dose 103%. Loading: (1) anterior: 70 cGy/fr; (2) posterior: 70 cGy/fr; (3) right lateral: 30 cGy/fr; (4) left lateral: 30 cGy/fr.

- *Special considerations.* The upper limit in very frail patients can be lowered to the level of the mid-sacroiliac joints. After 60 Gy, the boost dose to the prostate can be given through a direct perineal field. After prostatectomy, the dose to the prostatic area should not be above 60 Gy. Whole pelvis irradiation is often omitted.

13.7.3 Palliative irradiation of the pelvis

In very advanced cases which can lead to a frozen pelvis, palliative irradiation may be proposed to improve micturition, calm pain, and alleviate venous or lymphatic compression. A simple technique with AP–PA fields and moderate dose is advisable.

- *Position.* Supine with a fully distended bladder if possible.
- *Localization.* Marks on the anal margin.
- *Field margins.*

  upper limit: mid-sacroiliac point
  lower limit: lower border of the ischial tuberosities
  lateral limit: 1 cm outside the pelvic rim

- *Dose prescription.* The dose is 30 Gy in 10 fractions over 2 weeks.
- *Special considerations.* The limits of field can be adapted according to the clinical situation. Blocks can be positioned to protect organs at risk if needed. Dose and fractionation can be adapted to meet the clinical situation.

13.7.4 Preventive therapy for gynaecomastia

In cases of oestrogen treatment, gynaecomastia may be prevented by prior irradiation of the male breast tissue with an anterior field of 8×8 cm centred on the nipple to give 10 Gy in a single fraction or up to four fractions.

13.8 MORBIDITY

Acute morbidity may include early cystitis, urethritis or proctitis. Anti-inflammatory and antibiotic treatment may control these reactions. Late toxicity in 5% of radical treatments may include chronic cystitis with haematuria or radiation proctitis with rectorrhagia.

Urethral stricture may require dilatation. Impotence occurs in 30–50% of cases within five years after irradiation.

13.9 CHEMOTHERAPY

The results of chemotherapy for prostate cancer are disappointing. No cytotoxic agents are recommended for specific or adjuvant therapy.

Hormonal inhibitors of gonadotrophin secretion (leuprolide, etc.), however, are effective in the palliative treatment of advanced prostatic cancer.

14

Bladder

14.1 INCIDENCE AND RISK FACTORS

Bladder cancer represents approximately 2% of all malignant tumours in Western countries. The peak incidence occurs in the seventh decade of life. Accurate statistics are not available in most developing countries, but in Egypt bladder cancer is the first most common tumour in men and the second most common in women. In Zimbabwe, it is estimated to be the fourth most common malignancy in either sex.

There is a two- to sixfold increased risk of bladder cancer in cigarette smokers, and this risk increases in proportion to the number of cigarettes smoked. Analgesic abuse, for example with compounds containing phenacetin, also increases the risk of urothelial malignancy. Bladder cancer is an occupational hazard for those who may be exposed to aromatic amines such as benzidine and ß-naphthylamine, for example workers in the organic chemical industries and the paint, rubber or dye industries.

There is a close association between schistosomiasis and squamous cell carcinoma of the bladder in endemic areas such as Egypt and Central Africa.

14.2 PRESENTATION AND NATURAL HISTORY

Painless haematuria occurs in up to 75% of patients with bladder cancer. Microscopic haematuria also requires proper investigations as up to 22% of such patients have a urothelial malignancy. Extensive carcinoma *in situ* is frequently associated with dysuria and frequent urination in the absence of urinary infection.

In the presence of more advanced tumours, patients may present with a suprapubic mass, pelvic pain, oedema of the lower limbs secondary to lymphatic or venous occlusion, a malignant fistula into the vagina or the rectum, bladder outflow or rectal obstruction or uraemia from bilateral ureteric obstruction. Other patients present with symptoms of metastatic disease.

Death is usually due to uraemia, cachexia or haemorrhage.

14.3 HISTOPATHOLOGY

In the West, transitional cell carcinoma is the most common histological type, whereas squamous cell carcinoma constitutes up to 80% of bladder cancer in schistosomiasis-endemic areas. Adenocarcinoma of the bladder is uncommon and is thought to arise from the urachal remnant. Sarcoma of the bladder is rare.

14.4 INVESTIGATIONS

Urinary cytology may suggest the diagnosis of bladder cancer but an intravenous urogram is necessary in all cases. This may show the tumour as a filling defect in the bladder. The diagnosis is confirmed by cystoscopy and transurethral biopsy or resection of the suspected area with the patient under anaesthesia. The biopsy should be deep enough to enable assessment of possible muscle invasion, and other sites adjacent to and distant from the tumour should be biopsied to exclude the presence of carcinoma *in situ*, which has an influence on management and prognosis. Bimanual examination should be performed at the time of biopsy to assess the local and pelvic extent of the tumour.

Further staging and assessment of any extravesical tumour extensions and lymph node or organ involvement, as well as the status of the kidneys, may be done using ultrasound and computed tomographic scanning, where available. A complete blood count, renal function tests and biochemical profile should be completed and a chest radiograph performed.

14.5 STAGING AND PROGNOSIS

The TNM (1987) classification is recommended (Table 14.1).

The prognosis in bladder cancer is closely related to the tumour stage at diagnosis, but the patient's age and fitness also affect

Table 14.1 Classification of bladder cancer (UICC, 1987)

Stage	Description
Tis	Carcinoma *in situ*; 'flat tumour'
Ta	Non-invasive papillary carcinoma
T1	Tumour invades subepithelial connective tissue
T2	Tumour invades superficial muscle
T3a	Tumour invades deep muscle
T3b	Tumour invades perivesical fat
T4	Tumour invades any of the following: prostate, bowel, uterus, vagina, pelvis wall, abdominal wall
The suffix (m) indicates multiple tumours	
N0	No regional lymph node metastases
N1	Metastases in a single lymph node, ≤ 2 cm
N2	Metastases in a single lymph node, 2–5 cm, or multiple lymph nodes, none > 5 cm
N3	Metastases in a lymph node, > 5 cm
M0	No distant metastases
M1	Distant metastases

prognosis as they may influence the choice of treatment. In most developing countries, the majority of patients with bladder cancer present late with T3 to T4 invasive tumours. Invasion of the bladder wall is associated with a higher incidence of lymph node and distant metastases: 30% of patients with superficial muscle invasion and 60% with deep muscle invasion will have lymph node metastases. The median survival of patients with N1 disease is 13 months and is much worse for more advanced nodal disease. The expected survival in untreated invasive bladder cancer is less than 5% at two years, and up to 50% of patients with invasive disease die with metastatic cancer. Non-invasive (superficial) tumours or T1 lesions have a better prognosis and treatment by transurethral resection alone may be curative. Symptoms and signs which suggest bladder cancer should therefore be investigated promptly to ensure early diagnosis and better prognosis as disease progression is inevitable.

Transitional cell carcinoma has a better prognosis than squamous cell carcinoma, and younger patients treated with radical surgery do better than patients treated with radical radiotherapy alone.

The overall five-year survival rate following radical surgery for invasive bladder cancer is 15–30%. For low-grade T1 or T2 tumours, cure rates of up to 80% can be achieved. Following radical radiotherapy, the five-year survival for high-grade or multiple T1 tumours is around 50%, for T2 tumours it is 30–40% and for T3 and T4 it is 5–30%.

14.6 TREATMENT – CHOICE OF MODALITY

14.6.1 General considerations

In the West, bladder cancer has a peak incidence in the seventh decade of life, but in countries where schistosomiasis is endemic, younger patients are often seen. The patient's age and fitness are important considerations in the choice of treatment modality. Thus younger and fitter patients may undergo repeated cystoscopic resections for superficial tumours, with the attendant anaesthetic risks, or be suitable for radical cystectomy if they have carcinoma *in situ* or early (T2–T3) invasive cancer. In contrast elderly or unfit patients may be treated with intravesical chemotherapy for superficial tumours or radical radiotherapy for invasive cancer, with cystectomy reserved for salvage in suitable cases.

In developing countries, the available surgical skills, radiotherapy facilities or drugs also greatly influence the choice of treatment, in addition to the stage at presentation. Furthermore, cultural influence and limited knowledge make many suitable patients unwilling to accept cystectomy. Lack of supporting medical services may make the doctor reluctant to recommend cystectomy and urinary diversion, with its potential metabolic and infective complications.

14.6.2 Superficial bladder cancer, including T1 tumours

(a) Surgery

All cases require transurethral resection, both for staging and treatment. This may be curative for low-grade lesions. However, patients presenting with carcinoma *in situ*, multiple or high-grade tumours have a worse prognosis and should preferably have a cystectomy. If the prostatic urethra is involved, treatment is by a cystoprostatectomy. Transurethral resection alone is not adequate treatment for squamous cell carcinoma and it should be followed by cystectomy or radical radiotherapy.

The majority of recurrences occur within two years. A check cystoscopy should be done after three months and thereafter every six months until two years. If no recurrence is detected by that time, cystoscopy is then performed at yearly intervals. Intravesical chemotherapy may reduce recurrence rates.

(b) Intravesical chemotherapy

This may be used for carcinoma *in situ* not treated by immediate cystectomy and for multifocal papillary tumours not controlled by transurethral resection. The drugs are instilled into the bladder and left for two hours, during which time the patient is instructed to change position often to ensure maximum distribution of the drug inside the bladder. Drugs used include thiotepa, epodyl, mitomycin C and doxorubicin.

(c) External beam irradiation

This is not successful in controlling carcinoma *in situ* or other superficial bladder cancer. However, radical radiotherapy is moderately effective in grade 3 T1 lesions and up to 50% of patients may be controlled.

Interstitial and intracavitary irradiation for bladder cancer are best performed in specialized centres and are not generally recommended.

14.6.3 Invasive bladder cancer

Radical surgery and radical radiotherapy remain the two most effective treatment modalities for invasive bladder cancer. For reasons which include shortage of specialist surgeons and supporting health facilities, external beam radiotherapy is the most commonly used form of therapy in developing countries. In schistosomiasis-endemic areas, this means that treatment results are not as good since squamous cell carcinoma of the bladder responds poorly to radical radiotherapy compared with transitional cell carcinoma. Salvage cystectomy, if available, may improve survival.

(a) Surgery

Radical cystoprostatectomy in men or anterior exenteration in women is the treatment of choice. The procedure carries an operative mortality rate of 5–15%. Partial cystectomy is indicated in well-selected cases of histologically proven solitary primary tumours, ideally located in the upper part or posterior wall of the bladder. Contra-indications to this procedure include a tumour < 3 cm from the bladder neck, invasion of the prostate, carcinoma *in situ*, multiple or recurrent tumours, previous irradiation or small bladder volume.

(b) External beam radiotherapy

This can be given with curative intent in T2, T3N0M0 tumours when surgery is not indicated. It is recommended before partial cystectomy to prevent scar implant. Doses of 10 Gy in 3 fractions have been shown to be effective in this situation.

14.6.4 Palliative treatment

Patients with advanced bladder cancer frequently have severe pelvic pain. The physician should not hesitate to commence such patients on morphine while awaiting the effects of other measures such as pelvic irradiation. Haematuria or haemorrhage and anaemia are also common. Uraemia is best left untreated. Palliative radiotherapy may be given for relief of symptoms such as haematuria and pelvic pain in locally advanced tumours and metastatic disease, especially in bones.

14.7 RADIOTHERAPY TECHNIQUES

14.7.1 Radical irradiation

This is proposed for T2 N0 or small T3 N0 tumours which are deemed inoperable. The target volume is the whole bladder and pelvic lymph nodes including the common iliac nodes. The prescribed dose is 44 Gy to the pelvis and 64 Gy to the bladder and any extravesical extension. The technique is a four-field box technique with telecobalt.

- *Position*. Supine with a fully distended bladder when irradiating the whole pelvis and then an empty bladder.
- *Localization*. When irradiating only the bladder, a cystogram is mandatory. Contrast, e.g. 20 ml of contrast medium and 10 ml of air, is instilled into the bladder without draining residual urine.

Marks are placed on the anal margin. Barium enema may be used on the lateral film to visualize the rectum.

- *Field margins* (Figure 14.1).
  Pelvis:

  upper limit: at L5/S1 junction
  lower limit: at the inferior border of the obturator foramen which marks the floor of the true pelvis or lower if indicated by the cystogram
  lateral limits: 1 cm lateral to the bony pelvic wall
  anterior limit: 1 cm anterior to the pubic bone or 2 cm anterior to the bladder as seen on the cystogram (air) including extra-vesical extension
  posterior limit: between the middle and posterior thirds of the rectum or 2 cm behind the bladder as seen on the cystogram (dye)

  Bladder: irradiated in an empty condition with a four-field box technique with field sizes usually 9–11 cm × 9–11 cm:

  upper limit: 2 cm above the bladder as seen on the cystogram
  lower limit: same as pelvis
  anterior limit: same as pelvis
  posterior limit: same as pelvis
  lateral limit: 2 cm outside the lateral wall of the bladder

- *Beam modification.* Blocks to protect part of the small bowel and the head of the femur.
- *Dose prescription* (Figure 14.2). A dose of 44 Gy in 22 fractions over $4\frac{1}{2}$ weeks is prescribed to the pelvis, then an additional boost dose of 20 Gy is given to the bladder in 10 fractions over 2 weeks.
- *Special consideration.* An alternative is a three-field arrangement (one anterior, two lateral or two oblique lateral). A wedge filter must be used with two lateral and one anterior field.

14.7.2 Palliative irradiation

This is used to palliate symptoms such as haematuria or pain. The target volume is the bladder and extravesical extension. A simple technique with AP–PA fields and moderate dose is recommended.

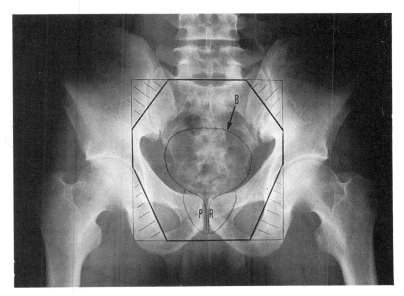

(a)

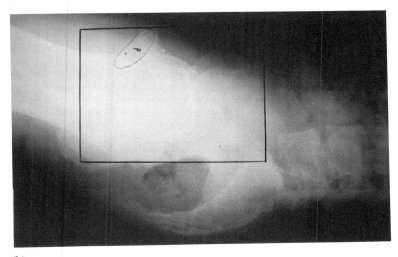

(b)

Figure 14.1 Radical irradiation. Outline of the field limits on a radiograph: (a) anterior field; (b) lateral field. P, pubic bone; PR, prostate; B, bladder.

- *Position.* Supine.
- *Localization.* Cystogram if needed, bladder empty.
- *Field margins.* The margins are 2 cm around the bladder or extravesical extension. Field sizes are usually 10–12 cm × 10–12 cm.
- *Dose prescription.* The dose is 30 Gy in 10 fractions over 2 weeks.
- *Special consideration.* The limits of the field can be adapted according to the clinical situation. Part of the pelvis can be included and blocks may be positioned if needed.

14.8 MORBIDITY

Early morbidity of radiation treatment includes radiation cystitis, tenesmus and diarrhoea. Mid-stream urine should be checked reg-

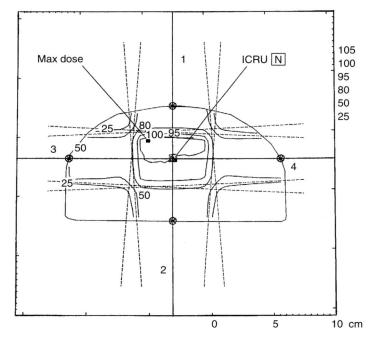

Figure 14.2 Radical irradiation. Isodose distribution for cobalt and SSD = 80 cm. ☐N☐ normalized on the 100% (ICRU) point; (■) maximum dose 102%. Loading: (1) anterior: 70 cGy/fr; (2) posterior: 70 cGy/fr; (3) right lateral: 30 cGy/fr; (4) left lateral: 30 cGy/fr.

ularly to exclude urinary infection. In severe acute reactions, treatment may need to be suspended for some days while appropriate treatments to improve symptoms are given.

The late effects of radical radiotherapy may include a contracted small volume bladder, bladder telangiectasia with haematuria and small bowel or rectal damage. Regular follow-up of patients is therefore necessary both to monitor response to treatment and detect recurrence early, and to treat appropriately any severe late complications of therapy. A check cystoscopy should be done three-monthly twice, then six-monthly until two years. Thereafter annual checks are adequate. Non-responding or relapsing patients may be selected for salvage cystectomy. The patient should also be seen by the radiotherapist every 3–6 months, preferably in a joint urology clinic.

15

Penis

15.1 INCIDENCE AND RISK FACTORS

Carcinoma of the penis is a rare tumour in Western countries, about 1–2 cases per 100 000 men per year, but the incidence is much higher in south east Asia, Africa and China, where it may account for 10–15% of genito-urinary malignancies. In high-incidence groups, the tumour appears to be related to phimosis and poor hygiene. Early circumcision greatly reduces the risk of the disease by facilitating personal hygiene and removal of smegma which is believed to be carcinogenic.

15.2 PRESENTATION AND NATURAL HISTORY

Penile carcinoma usually presents as an ulcer or exophytic lesion on the glans or coronal sulcus. There is often wide surface extension before deeper extension occurs to the urethra or corpora cavernosa. The differential diagnosis includes syphilis, chancroid, lymphogranuloma venereum and granuloma inguinale. Any suspicious lesion of the penis should be biopsied. Associated phimosis is common, as are secondary infection and foul odour. Urethral obstruction is unusual. Inguinal nodes are palpable in many cases, but contain tumour in only about 50% due to the high incidence of inflammatory processes causing lymphadenopathy. The use of antibiotics for several weeks before making a decision on the status of the nodes was previously recommended, but with better ultrasound and fine-needle aspiration cytology, it is now possible to resolve the issue more speedily.

Slow, loco-regional progression is characteristic of this disease. Distant metastases are rare but, when they occur, the commonest sites are lungs and bone. Since distant metastases are uncommon in this tumour, the weakness, weight loss and fatigue not uncommonly seen in advanced cases are more often a result of chronic infection and suppuration.

15.3 HISTOPATHOLOGY

Premalignant conditions of the penis include condylomata acuminata, Bowen's disease, erythroplasia of Queyrat and leucoplasia. Erythroplasia of Queyrat is carcinoma *in situ* of the glans and presents as a red, velvety lesion. Some patients with penile warts have developed penile carcinoma. Thus, these lesions should always be treated actively, generally by surgery. Most penile carcinomas are well-differentiated squamous cell carcinomas. Anaplasia has been described as associated with a worse prognosis but there is conflicting evidence regarding this.

15.4 INVESTIGATIONS

Clinical examination is essential for a good staging. Routine investigations should include:

- radiographs of the chest;
- a swab from any discharging lesion and a mid-stream urine sample for culture and sensitivity; and
- serological tests for syphilis.

15.5 STAGING AND PROGNOSIS

The staging system most commonly used for carcinoma of the penis is the TNM system (Table 15.1). An alternative is the Jackson staging system.

Staging in carcinoma of the penis is closely related to prognosis. Most T1 lesions are cured but few T3 and very few T4, N3 or M1. The Jackson system has the advantage that it relates to operability: most stage I and many stage II are cured, fewer stage III and very few stage IV.

Size is also important. Tumours under 2 cm on the distal third have an 80% cure rate, whereas only 20% of such tumours on the

Table 15.1 Classification of penis carcinoma

Method	Stage	Description
TNM	T1	Invasion of subepithelial connective tissue
(UICC,	T2	Invasion of corpus spongiosum or cavernosum
1987)	T3	Invasion of urethra or prostate
	T4	Invasion of other structures
	N0	No nodal metastasis
	N1	Single superficial inguinal node involved
	N2	Multiple or bilateral superficial inguinal node involvement
	N3	Deep inguinal or pelvic node involvement
	M0	No distant metastasis
	M1	Distant metastasis
Jackson	I	Tumour confined to glans or prepuce
	II	Tumour extending on to shaft of penis
	III	Tumour with operable inguinal metastases
	IV	Tumour with inoperable metastases

proximal third are cured. If regional nodes are tumour-free, there is an excellent (85–90%) cure rate, whereas patients with involved nodes have only 40–50% long-term survival.

15.6 TREATMENT – CHOICE OF MODALITY

15.6.1 Radical treatment

Since the disease is generally localized on presentation, most cases should be treated radically. Treatment decisions are based on the stage, site, age and psychological status of the patient. The need to retain sexual function and the ability to micturate upright are of paramount importance in young men. Most commonly, the management involves surgery and/or radiotherapy.

(a) Surgery

Surgical management involves amputation of part or the whole of the penis. Frozen section is recommended, with a 2 cm clear resection margin. Some superficial penile lesions can be treated using an ND:YAG laser.

Mobile involved inguinal nodes should be treated by lymphade-nectomy and post-operative radiotherapy. The management of clini-cally negative nodes is more controversial. We know that up to 20% of clinically negative nodes contain tumour. On the other hand, prophylactic groin dissection is associated with some morbidity: infection, wound dehiscence and chronic lymphoedema. In Western countries, therefore, a T1 tumour with negative groin nodes can be managed by a 'wait and watch' policy. However, where follow-up is likely to be poor, as in many developing countries, or with a more advanced primary tumour, it is best to opt for prophylactic groin dissection.

(b) Radiotherapy

Radiotherapy has the major advantage of preserving the penis. Since oedema induced by radiotherapy may lead to urethral ob-struction, it is often necessary to perform a dorsal slit or circum-cision prior to starting irradiation. There are three ways of administering radiation in this situation and the choice will de-pend on the site, size, depth of invasion and the stage of the tumour.

1. Superficial radiotherapy: 100–250 V X-rays may be adequate for small superficial carcinomas, with a margin of at least 0.5 cm around the tumour. A dose of 50–55 Gy/15–20 fr/3–4 weeks is given or the equivalent.
2. Megavoltage irradiation: This is the non-surgical technique of choice for all infiltrating tumours or tumours involving nodes. Prophylactic groin irradiation is an unresolved issue and has not been proven to be of benefit in Western countries. However, with bulky tumours or tumours which involve the corpora cavernosa or are poorly differentiated or in patients where good follow-up is unlikely, prophylactic groin irradiation should be given if a groin dissection cannot be performed. Clinically involved groin nodes should be treated by lymphadenectomy and post-operative radiotherapy.
3. Implantation: Iridium-192 is highly flexible and suitable for single-plane implantation, especially for small tumours spread-ing circumferentially without deep infiltration. A dose of 60 Gy is given over four days.

(c) Chemotherapy

Chemotherapy is little used in the radical management of penile cancer, although it is increasingly used in relapsed cases in Western countries. The most effective cytotoxic agents against penile carcinoma are methotrexate, bleomycin and *cis*-platin. Occasional complete remissions are seen which may last over a year, but in general response rates are disappointing.

15.6.2 Palliative treatment

Palliative radiotherapy may be used for incurable tumours causing symptoms, especially pain or discharge. A standard dose for palliative radiotherapy is 50 Gy/25 fr/5 weeks. It may be desirable to use a shorter course, e.g. 40 Gy/15 fr/3 weeks, but, with the degree of hypoxia and sepsis commonly seen in these tumours, more fractionated treatment is more effective. Antibiotics and antiseptics should be given concomitantly.

Many patients with penile carcinoma present late, especially in developing countries, with incurable primary tumour or inoperable nodes, causing pain, ulceration, sepsis and lymphoedema of the scrotum and extremities. Radiotherapy to the primary or nodes can relieve ulceration or pain. If the pain does not respond to radiation, anaesthetic measures may be used. Leg lymphoedema may respond to bandaging, elevation at night, dexamethasone or radiotherapy to the groin, but may persist despite these measures. These patients frequently require morphine, preferably given four-hourly, orally, in tablet form. Since the terminal phase may be prolonged, both the patients and their families may require considerable support and counselling.

15.7 RADIOTHERAPY TECHNIQUES

15.7.1 Radical megavoltage irradiation alone

This technique is indicated in case of infiltrating tumours (stage T2). The target volume is the whole glans and part of the shaft depending on its infiltration by the tumour. The prescribed dose is 60 Gy. The technique involves two parallel opposed fields with the penis fully bolused.

- *Position.* Supine with the penis maintained in a vertical position using a wax bolus.
- *Localization.* By clinical assessment.
- *Field margins.* All the limits are at the fall-off 1.5 cm around the penis except the proximal limit which is 2 cm below any detectable tumour in the shaft.
- *Beam modification.* A two-wax-block bolus is made and tailored to the penis and the tumour. The telecobalt unit is tilted at 90° and 270° to produce horizontal beams. The average field size is 5–7 cm × 5–7 cm.
- *Dose prescription.* The dose to the penis is 60 Gy in 30 fractions over 6 weeks.

15.7.2 Post-operative irradiation of the groin

This is performed after inguinal lymphadenectomy when metastatic nodes are found by the pathologist. Irradiation starts after full healing of the scar which can take 4–8 weeks. The target volume is the inguinal area, with a depth varying from 2 to 3 cm. The prescribed dose is 50 Gy. The technique involves one direct field with telecobalt.

- *Position.* Supine, with legs angled out; scrotum and abdominal wall can be retracted out of the field if necessary.
- *Localization.* Performed clinically. A radiograph film is taken to check the position of the head of the femur, usually in the centre of the field. Care should be taken not to overdose the coxofemoral joint and the upper extremity of the femur.
- *Field margins.* The field sizes are usually 8–11 cm × 7–10 cm. The centre of the field is on the femoral artery at the level of the crural arcade.
- *Dose prescription.* The dose per fraction is 200 cGy calculated at 3 cm. The total dose is 50 Gy in 25 fractions over 5 weeks.
- *Special consideration.* Blocks can be used to shield the inner part of the field. In very thin patients, the dose can be calculated at 2 cm or even at the given dose point (0.5 cm). If the nodes are not removed, a total dose of up to 64 Gy can be used. If available, electrons are very useful to irradiate this inguinal area sometimes in a mixed beam with cobalt (one-third of the dose) and 6–12 MeV electrons (two-thirds of the dose).

15.8   MORBIDITY

15.8.1 Early morbidity

An early reaction to radiotherapy seen in many patients is a brisk skin reaction with swelling of the subcutaneous tissues of the shaft. Although uncomfortable, this usually resolves within a few weeks. Many patients also develop burning dysuria which may result in urinary retention. A catheter may prevent this problem.

15.8.2 Late morbidity

Late complications include fibrosis with atrophy. Strictures and meatal stenosis can occur but are dealt with by dilatation. Ulceration and necrosis of the glans or of the skin of the shaft are rare complications. Lymphoedema of the lower limb has been reported following radiotherapy but is usually associated with lymphatic involvement by tumour. Erectile function is maintained in most patients.

16

Kidney

16.1 INCIDENCE AND RISK FACTORS

Carcinoma of the kidney represents approximately 2% of all malignancies. The peak incidence occurs in the fifth to seventh decades, with a male to female ratio range of 1.5–2.1.

Cigarette smoking increases the risk of developing renal cell carcinoma. Increased incidence is also seen among workers exposed to asbestos and cadmium, and among leather tanners and shoe workers. Analgesic abuse, especially analgesic compounds containing phenacetin, phenazone and caffeine, is associated with an increased risk, particularly of cancer of the renal pelvis. Squamous cell carcinoma of the renal pelvis is usually associated with chronic urinary tract inflammation or infection, such as schistosomiasis.

16.2 PRESENTATION AND NATURAL HISTORY

The majority of patients present with flank pain and haematuria. In the early stages, the haematuria is usually painless. The classic triad of pain, haematuria and the presence of a flank mass occurs in only about 10–20% of patients and usually indicates advanced disease. Approximately 30% will present with symptoms and signs of distant metastases, commonly to the lungs, but also to bones, liver and brain.

Many patients with renal carcinoma develop systematic manifestations. These include hypochromic anaemia, weight loss, hypercalcaemia, hypertension, pyrexia, non-metastatic hepatic dysfunction and cachexia. Other symptoms include polycythaemia, neuromyopathy and amyloidosis. Renal cell carcinoma has thus aptly been called the 'great imitator'. Some of the non-metastatic manifestations may resolve when the renal cancer is resected. Death is usually due to haemorrhage, cachexia, hypercalcaemia, organ failure or a combination of these factors.

16.3 HISTOPATHOLOGY

The most common cancer of the kidney is renal cell carcinoma, also called adenocarcinoma of the kidney or hypernephroma (95% of renal tumours). The histological subtypes are:

- clear cell type: 75%
- granular cell type: 15%
- sarcomatoid type: 10%.

Carcinoma of the renal pelvis accounts for the remaining 5%, and 90% of these are transitional cell carcinoma. Squamous cell carcinoma (7%) and adenocarcinoma constitute the remainder.

16.4 INVESTIGATIONS

Intravenous urography is usually the initial investigation but may appear normal despite the presence of a small tumour. It also provides information about the location and function of the contralateral kidney, which is essential information when contemplating surgery.

Ultrasound examination provides both staging and diagnostic information. It will distinguish between a solid or cystic renal mass and demonstrate extra-renal extension of the tumour, adrenal or lymph node involvement, and infiltration of adjacent organs. It can also assess renal vein and inferior vena cava involvement. Aspiration of solid renal masses during ultrasound examination is not recommended because of the risk of tumour implantation in the needle track.

Computed tomography with contrast enhancement is less readily available in developing countries but is the single most informative diagnostic technique. It can identify small renal masses as well as demonstrate extra-renal extensions and involvement of vessels, lymph nodes and adjacent viscera.

A renal arteriogram is useful in evaluating a small indeterminate renal mass, and in showing the number and position of the renal arteries, which aids surgical removal. Arteriography can also be

Table 16.1 Classification of kidney cancer (UICC, 1987)

Stage	Description
TX	Primary tumour cannot be assessed
T1	Tumour $\leq$ 2.5 cm, limited to kidney
T2	Tumour $>$ 2.5 cm, limited to kidney
T3a	Tumour invades adrenal gland or perinephric tissues but not beyond Gerota's fascia
T3b	Tumour grossly extends into renal vein(s) or vena cava
T4	Tumour invades beyond Gerota's fascia, e.g. muscle, bowel or liver
NX	Regional lymph nodes cannot be assessed
N0	No regional lymph node metastasis
N1	Metastasis in a single lymph node, $\leq$ 2 cm
N2	Metastasis in a single lymph node, 2–5 cm, or multiple lymph nodes, none $>$ 5 cm
N3	Metastasis in a lymph node, $>$ 5 cm
MX	Distant metastasis cannot be assessed
M0	No distant metastasis
M1	Distant metastasis

used for pre-operative embolization of vascular tumours or for palliative embolization. However, non-invasive methods of investigation are now generally preferred.

Baseline investigations should include complete blood count, biochemical profile, liver function tests, chest radiograph and skeletal survey or bone scan.

16.5 STAGING AND PROGNOSIS

The TNM classification is recommended (Table 16.1).

Favourable prognostic features of renal cell carcinoma are small tumours less than 5 cm in size without extra-renal extension, non-invasion of vessels, and clear-cell or granular-cell type histology. The sarcomatoid type has a bad prognosis. Squamous cell carcinoma of the renal pelvis also has a poor prognosis.

The presence of distant metastases is the single worst prognostic feature with 0% five-year survival. However, patients with solitary pulmonary metastases (1–3% of cases) have a 30–50% five-year survival rate when treated by nephrectomy and pulmonary resection. Lymphatic metastases are also a bad feature, with 0–30% five-year survival.

The best survival is obtained in fit patients with early stage disease who are able to undergo radical surgery. Radical nephrectomy gives an overall five-year survival of 30–50%, but for T1 and T2 tumours it results in a 60–80% five-year survival. Patients with more extensive tumours have a worse prognosis, with survival figures of around 10% for T3 and T4 tumours. For renal pelvis tumours, the best results are achieved with superficial tumours, and the overall five-year survival rate is 50–60%.

The major risks of radical surgery include haemorrhage, bowel injury and sepsis. Radiotherapy may also cause damage to the small bowel and liver, which may be fatal in some cases.

Regular follow-up, initially at 2–3 monthly intervals, is necessary for the early detection and treatment of any complications of treatment. Furthermore, the few patients who subsequently develop solitary lung or brain metastases may still be cured. Attention should also be given to the possibility of new primary tumours arising in other parts of the urothelium, especially bladder cancers.

16.6 TREATMENT – CHOICE OF MODALITY

16.6.1 Radical treatment

Treatment modalities employed in managing renal cancer include surgery, radiotherapy, angio-infarction, hormone therapy, immunotherapy and chemotherapy. The last three modalities are all relatively ineffective. The choice of treatment modality will depend on the tumour stage at diagnosis, the age and general condition of the patient and whether metastases are present.

(a) Surgery

The only curative treatment for renal cancer is radical nephrectomy, which involves removal of the intact kidney within Gerota's fascia, and of the adrenal and the regional lymph nodes. Embolization of the tumour may be used before surgery to reduce vascularity. If the tumour extends into the vena cava, partial or total resection of a portion of the vena cava may be required.

In developing countries where the majority of patients are diagnosed with advanced disease, palliative nephrectomy is often needed to control symptoms of pain, haemorrhage, hypercalcaemia or hypertension or to treat the post-embolization syndrome (pain, ileus, sepsis). Palliative embolization via the renal artery may be performed in patients unfit for major surgery or when distant metastases are present.

Solitary metastases in the lung or brain should be resected, when the primary tumour is operable, as long-term survival can be achieved. Post-operative radiotherapy, 40–60 Gy/20–30 fr/4–6 weeks, is usually given following such resections. Nephrectomy should not be performed for the sole purpose of inducing regression of metastases as this rarely occurs, if ever.

(b) Radiotherapy

Radiotherapy has a limited role in the definitive management of renal cancer. Following radical nephrectomy, post-operative radiotherapy may improve local control, especially for T3 and T4 tumours. However, prospective studies have shown no survival benefits. The usual radiation dose is 40–50 Gy/20–25 fr/4–5 weeks given to a field covering the renal fossa, tumour bed and the paraortic and paracaval lymph nodes (medial field border 2 cm beyond vertebral bodies). Usually parallel opposed fields on a megavoltage machine are used. A typical field size is 14×13 cm. The upper border of the field is approximately the T11/12 junction and the lower border approximately the L4/5 junction.

(c) Other modalities: hormone therapy and immunotherapy

Progestogens, e.g. medroxyprogesterone acetate and anti-oestrogens, e.g. tamoxifen, as well as other hormones have been used in the treatment of metastatic renal cell carcinoma or as an adjuvant but are mostly ineffective. Their routine use is not recommended. Similarly, immunotherapy using agents such as BCG, interferon or interleukin-2, although of interest, is still in the experimental stages and is not yet generally applicable.

16.6.2 Palliative treatment

Palliative radiotherapy is most useful for relief of pain from bony metastases, but gives good symptomatic relief at all metastatic sites. A typical dose is 30 Gy/10 fr/2 weeks. When the primary tumour is inoperable, intermediate high-dose radiotherapy, 40–50 Gy/20–25 fr/4–5 weeks, may relieve pain and haematuria in about 50% of patients.

The natural history of renal cancer indicates that pain control, alleviation of haematuria, blood transfusions for anaemia, treatment of hypercalcaemia and pinning of the long bones to prevent pathological fractures are the more common measures that will improve the quality of life for the patient with advanced disease.

17

Testicle

17.1 INCIDENCE AND RISK FACTORS

Testicular germ-cell tumours represent approximately 1% of malignancies in men in developed countries, where their incidence is rising at an alarming rate. The cause of this rise is unknown. There would appear to be a racial link to the aetiology since in mixed societies such as the USA, the increased incidence appears confined to Caucasians. Maldescent of the testis is a known predisposing factor, increasing the risk of this tumour by five- to tenfold over the risk in the population as a whole, and there is a similar level of increased risk in brothers of affected men. The premalignant phase of carcinoma *in situ* can only be recognized reliably following a testicular biopsy. The main subjects at risk of testicular germ-cell tumours are those 20–45 years old; the rarity of the tumour makes screening programmes impracticable.

17.2 PRESENTATION AND NATURAL HISTORY

Ninety-five per cent of men with germ-cell tumours have an overt testicular primary tumour, with the remainder presenting with evidence of metastatic disease and a very small primary tumour; uncommonly, the germ-cell tumour may arise at a primary site which is extragonadal, such as the anterior mediastinum or the pineal region.

The typical finding on examination of a testicular primary tumour is that the tumour is hard and painless, although a small proportion of patients do have discomfort. The differential diagnosis includes epididymo-orchitis, tuberculosis, epididymitis, gumma of the testis, torsion, hydrocele or hernia.

Manifestations of metastatic disease at presentation include backache from retroperitoneal node metastases or dyspnoea, cough and occasionally haemoptysis from lung metastases. The non-seminomatous tumours may secrete alpha-fetoprotein (AFP) or human chorionic gonadotrophin (hCG) which can be identified in the serum by radioimmunoassay or in the case of hCG in urine by pregnancy testing. Some patients may present with gynaecomastia.

Delay of diagnosis is common, usually as a result of the patient's delay in seeking medical advice. It is, therefore, appropriate to encourage public education campaigns with regard to the possibility that a testicular abnormality in a young man may represent a curable tumour. In the UK, an average delay of 3–4 months occurs between the patient noticing an abnormality and the diagnosis being established by orchidectomy. A longer delay is associated with a higher incidence of advanced metastatic disease.

17.3 HISTOPATHOLOGY

The majority are germ-cell tumours which are divided into carcinomas and teratomas. The pathological classifications of these tumours are shown in Table 17.1.

17.4 INVESTIGATIONS

The diagnosis is confirmed by inguinal orchidectomy which allows withdrawal of the testis intact. The dense membrane of the tunica albuginea tends to limit the local extension; however, this barrier is usually breached when a scrotal orchidectomy is performed and this may allow local recurrence.

Following histological confirmation of the diagnosis, investigations should include a physical examination directed towards detection of a retroperitoneal mass or supraclavicular lymph node metastasis. Where feasible, the tumour markers AFP and ß-hCG should be assayed since a sequential rise following orchidectomy is indicative of metastases. Further investigation of retroperitoneal nodes may involve ultrasound scans, computed tomographic scan or lymphography. Supradiaphragmatic metastasis from seminoma is extremely rare in the absence of abdominal node involvement and a plain chest radiograph allows appropriate staging. In non-seminomas, small lung metastases are common and lung tomo-

Table 17.1 WHO classification of testicular tumours (UICC, 1987)

Stage	Description

I	Germ-cell tumours
	A Tumours of one histological type:
	  1. Seminoma
	  2. Spermatocytic seminoma
	  3. Embryonal carcinoma
	  4. Yolk sac tumour (embryonal carcinoma, infantile type, endodermal sinus tumour)
	  5. Polyembryoma
	  6. Choriocarcinoma
	  7. Teratomas: (a) mature; (b) immature; (c) with malignant transformation
	B Tumours of more than one histological type:
	  1. Embryonal carcinoma and teratoma (teratocarcinoma)
	  2. Choriocarcinoma and any other types (specify type)
	  3. Other combinations (specify)

II	Sex cord/stromal tumours
III	Tumours containing both germ cell and sex cord/stromal elements
IV	Miscellaneous tumours
V	Lymphoid and haematopoietic tumours
IV	Secondary tumours
VII	Tumours of collecting ducts, rete, epididymis, spermatic cord, capsule, supporting structures and appendages

graphy or axial computed tomography will detect metastases in the 10–20% of patients whose chest radiographs are normal.

The first-level nodes are in the paraortic region, but this pattern of lymphatic dissemination may be disturbed in patients who have had previous inguinal surgery or who have locally advanced primary tumours. Other common sites of involvement for non-seminoma include lung fields and the supradiaphragmatic lymph nodes, but involvement of other organs is relatively uncommon except for pure trophoblastic tumours (choriocarcinomas) which progress rapidly and disseminate widely to other organs, especially including the liver and brain.

17.5 STAGING AND PROGNOSIS

The 1987 TNM staging of testicular tumours is illustrated in Table 17.2. Although it is useful to describe the extent of the primary

Table 17.2 TNM staging for testicular cancer (UICC, 1987)

Stage	Description
pTis	Intratubular
pT1	Testis and rete testis
pT2	Beyond tunica albuginea or into epididymis
pT3	Spermatic cord
pT4	Scrotum
N1	Single, $\leq$ 2 cm
N2	Single 2–5 cm, multiple $\leq$ 5 cm
N3	> 5 cm
M	Distant metastasis

Table 17.3 RMH (Royal Marsden Hospital) staging classification

Stage		Description
I	M	Rising post-orchidectomy markers only
II		Abdominal lymphadenopathy
	A	< 2 cm
	B	2–5 cm
	C	> 5 cm
III		Supradiaphragmatic lymphadenopathy
	O	No abdominal disease
	ABC	Abdominal node size as in stage II
IV		Extralymphatic metastases
	1.1	$\leq$ 3 lung metastases
	1.2	> 3 lung metastases all < 2 cm diameter
	1.3	> 3 lung metastases, of which one or more > 2 cm
	H +	Liver involvement

tumour, it is not commonly used internationally to describe metastatic disease and a more popular system is the Royal Marsden Hospital staging in which stage II represents retroperitoneal nodes, stage III represents supradiaphragmatic nodes and stage IV represents extranodal involvement (Table 17.3). It can be seen that the volume of disease, an important prognostic determinant, defines subdivisions of stage II and stage IV.

Non-seminomatous tumours are much more likely to present with metastatic disease and also metastases are more likely to have spread beyond retroperitoneal nodes.

Table 17.4 Prognosis of testicular cancer in the UK

	Main treatment post-orchidectomy	Proportion surviving
Teratomas		
Stage I	Surveillance/chemotherapy	98%
Stage II/III/IV	Chemotherapy	85%
Seminomas		
Stage I	Radiotherapy	98%
Stage II	Radiotherapy	95%
Stage III/IV	Chemotherapy	85%

The prognosis of germ-cell tumours of the testis is profoundly influenced by treatment, and, especially in the last two decades, the development of effective combination chemotherapy has dramatically improved the outlook for patients with advanced non-seminoma. The prognosis relating to clinical staging is presented in Table 17.4. Particularly adverse subgroups of non-seminoma include those with mediastinal primaries, trophoblastic tumours (choriocarcinomas) with high hCG levels, brain metastases or multiple (> 20) lung metastases, and there is also a slightly worse outlook in patients over 30 years old.

In seminoma, there are few established prognostic factors apart from stage. Those with histological evidence of a non-seminomatous component, or with raised serum AFP, should be treated as for non-seminomas.

17.6 TREATMENT – CHOICE OF MODALITY

Treatment is related to the histological subtype of germ-cell tumour and to the stage at presentation.

17.6.1 Stage I seminoma

A small proportion, 15–20%, of patients with clinical stage I seminoma will have subclinical metastases in retroperitoneal lymph nodes. The rarity of more widespread subclinical dissemination and the extreme radiosensitivity of seminoma make a policy of adjuvant retroperitoneal irradiation very logical. The relapse rate should be less than 5% following this treatment.

17.6.2 Stage II seminoma

Retroperitoneal node metastases up to 10 cm in diameter can be adequately treated and cured by radiotherapy. A high cure rate depends on very accurate radiological imaging, and larger tumours are treated with platinum-based chemotherapy in many centres. Where chemotherapy is not available, radiotherapy of bulky stage II seminoma should be supplemented by adjuvant radiotherapy to supradiaphragmatic nodes in the mediastinum and supraclavicular fossae.

17.6.3 Stage III/IV seminoma

The main line of treatment is platinum-based chemotherapy, since the cure rate using radiotherapy alone is less than 10%, whereas it is 80–90% with chemotherapy.

17.6.4 Stage I non-seminoma

Where expert radiological and chemical pathology facilities are available, policies of close surveillance have been developed for the management of patients with clinical stage I non-seminoma, but these require a regular attendance with assay of serum concentrations of AFP and hCG and regular computed tomographic scanning. These policies have demonstrated that even with very careful initial staging, some 30% of patients will relapse, with the most common relapse site being the retroperitoneal lymph nodes.

A second approach to stage I non-seminoma is to perform a retroperitoneal lymph node dissection which provides accurate information about staging and usually prevents the risk of abdominal node recurrence. In patients with pathologically normal retroperitoneal nodes the risk of relapse is less than 10%, but documented nodal involvement indicates a 35–70% risk of subsequent relapse depending on the extent of the lymphadenectomy. This risk may indicate that adjuvant platinum-based combination chemotherapy should be used.

A third approach to clinical stage I non-seminoma has been adjuvant retroperitoneal lymph node irradiation; however, these tumours are less sensitive than seminomas and a higher dose is required to prevent nodal recurrence. All methods of managing

Table 17.5 Chemotherapy combinations for testicular tumours

BEP	VAB-6
Cis-platin	Vinblastine
Etoposide	Cyclophosphamide
Bleomycin	Actinomycin-D
	Bleomycin
	Cis-platin

stage I non-seminoma should be associated with a cure rate of more than 90%.

17.6.5 Metastatic testicular non-seminoma

The mainstay of treatment is platinum-based combination chemotherapy, the most common schedule employing bleomycin, etoposide and *cis*-platin (Table 17.5). Radiotherapy has a limited role in the radical treatment of metastatic non-seminoma but can offer useful palliation in very moderate doses.

17.6.6 Palliative treatment

The great majority of testicular tumours are treated with curative intent. For patients relapsing after radiotherapy, combination chemotherapy will usually offer a curative option. For patients in whom chemotherapy has failed and with extensive disease beyond the possibility of cure with radical radiotherapy, palliation of symptoms can be achieved with moderate radiation doses and simple techniques, since both seminomas and non-seminomas are radiosensitive.

17.7 RADIOTHERAPY TECHNIQUES

17.7.1 Radical irradiation of a stage I seminoma

Irradiation is performed after orchidectomy and a complete work-up. The aim is to perform an elective radical irradiation of the lumbo-iliac lymph nodes. The target volume is the paraortic and ipsilateral pelvic lymph nodes. The prescribed dose is 27 Gy with fractions of 180 cGy. The technique is a 'dogleg' technique involving two parallel opposed fields with telecobalt.

- *Position.* Supine for both the anterior and the posterior field with patient's arm by his side.
- *Localization.* Marks on the inguinal scar of orchidectomy can be used if its irradiation is desired. Lymphangiography if performed in the work-up is very useful to localize the retroperitoneal lymph nodes. A mark on the testis may help to calculate the scattered dose to this critical organ. An intravenous urogram allows identification of the kidneys.
- *Field margins* (Figure 17.1).
  Anterior and posterior fields:

    upper limit: lower border of D11
    lower limit: lower border of the obturator foramen
    lateral limits: 1 cm lateral to the transverse apophysis of the vertebra to include all the lumbo-aortic lymph nodes with a safety margin. The field width is usually 8–10 cm. The width is

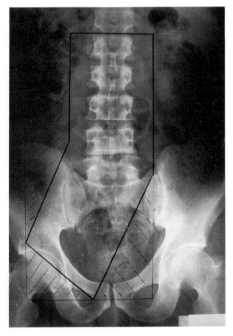

Figure 17.1 Radical iradiation. Outline of the field limits on a radiograph.

slightly smaller in the pelvis where only the ipsilateral pelvic nodes are irradiated.

- *Beam modifications.* Ideally, this complex field is created with custom-made blocks in cerobend alloy. It is possible also to use square and triangular lead shielding to shape the field and protect critical organs in the abdomen and the pelvis. The head of the femur must be shielded. The contralateral testis can be protected from scattered irradiation by a 1 cm lead cup.
- *Dose prescription.* The dose is prescribed on the midline of the lumbo-aortic region. The dose per fraction is 180 cGy ideally given each session through the anterior and posterior fields. The total dose is 27 Gy in 15 fractions over 3 weeks.
- *Special considerations.* The target volume can include the renal hilar nodes on the ipsilateral side. An intravenous urogram is important to delineate accurately the limits of such a field. The lower border may be extended to include the inguinal nodes in patients who have previously had inguinal or scrotal surgery. Scrotal irradiation may be indicated in patients whose locally advanced primary tumour had involved scrotal skin or if there had been a scrotal incision. In such cases the scrotum can be irradiated with photon energies of the order of 200–300 kV by a separate direct field matched to the inferior border of the dogleg using a lead cut-out. The length of this dogleg field may require treatment at extended FSD at the cost of a reduced dose rate.

In some situations, according to the treatment table design, the anterior field is applied with the patient supine and the posterior field with the patient in the prone position with the neck extended. An alternative to the dogleg field is to use two separate and matched fields to cover the paraortic nodes and the iliac nodes. The fields are equally weighted with the dose specified and prescribed at the midplane. The separation is at the level of the lower border of L5 and a 2–3 cm skin gap is calculated to avoid overlapping of the two fields.

For stage II seminoma the dogleg is treated to 27 Gy and then involved nodes are boosted by 6–10 Gy in 3–5 fractions over 3–5 days, with dose of 200 cGy per fraction. For non-seminomatous tumours the adjuvant dose in stage I is 40 Gy in 20 fractions over 4 weeks with boost of 6 Gy on involved nodes.

18

Hodgkin's disease

18.1 INCIDENCE AND RISK FACTORS

The annual incidence is approximately 4 per 100 000 in developed countries. However, it is one of the commonest cancers of young adults with a second peak of incidence at about age 55. There are striking geographic variations of age-specific incidence, with childhood Hodgkin's disease more frequent in less developed countries. At almost all ages, men have a greater incidence than women. No risk factors have been firmly established.

18.2 PRESENTATION AND NATURAL HISTORY

The presenting finding is most often a painless enlargement of peripheral lymph nodes, usually in the neck. Mediastinal involvement may often occur. As the disease becomes more advanced, splenic and paraortic extension occur. Approximately one-quarter of patients (but often higher proportions in developing countries) present with constitutional symptoms such as fevers, night sweats or weight loss. Extranodal involvement is rare at the time of initial presentation. However, as the disease progresses, numerous sites of involvement, such as bone, liver and lungs, may be seen.

18.3 HISTOPATHOLOGY

A biopsy is mandatory for diagnosis and will show Reed–Sternberg cells. The Rye and Lukes classification (1966) distinguishes four major groups:

1. lymphocytic predominance: 5%
2. nodular sclerosis: 50% with different subtypes mainly in young individuals
3. mixed cellularity: 35%
4. lymphocytic depletion: 10%.

The proportion may vary from one country to another.

18.4 INVESTIGATIONS

After the node biopsy which gives the positive diagnosis a careful work-up is mandatory, including:

1. a detailed clinical history, recording duration and the presence or absence of fever, unexplained sweating and its severity, and unexplained weight loss;
2. physical examination with special attention to all node-bearing areas, including Waldeyer's ring and determination of the size of the liver and spleen;
3. laboratory methods:
    (a) complete blood count including erythrocytic sedimentation rate;
    (b) evaluation of liver function: alkaline phosphatase, γGT levels;
    (c) evaluation of renal function; and
    (d) levels of serum uric acid, fibrinogen, blood iron, LDH;
4. radiological studies including:
    (a) chest: posterior–anterior
    (b) chest and abdominal computed tomographic scan if possible; and
    (c) bilateral lower extremity lymphogram in some cases;
5. staging laparotomy: now rarely performed because of better clinical staging; and
6. bone marrow biopsy in the presence of general symptoms or stage III–IV disease

18.5 STAGING AND PROGNOSIS

The Ann Arbor staging classification is commonly used (Table 18.1). The staging includes substaging into A and B categories. A

Table 18.1 Classification of Hodgkin's disease (Ann Arbor, 1970)

Stage	Definition	Five-year survival (%)
I	Involvement of a single lymph node region or a single extralymphatic organ or site (I_e)	95
II	Involvement of two or more lymph node regions (number to be stated) on the same side of the diaphragm (II) or localized involvement of extralymphatic organs or sites and/or one or more lymph node regions on the same side of the diaphragm (II_e)	70
III	Involvement of lymph node regions on both sides of the diaphragm (III) which may also be accompanied by localized involvement of extralymphatic organs or sites (III_e) or by involvement of the spleen (III_S) or both (III_{es})	60
IV	Diffuse or disseminated involvement of one or more extralymphatic organs or tissues with or without associated lymph node enlargement. The reasons for classifying the patient as stage IV are identified further by defining sites by means of the following symbols: N = lymph node; H = liver; M = marrow; P = pleura; S = spleen; L = lung; O = bone; D = skin	50

means the absence of constitutional symptoms; B means the presence of constitutional symptoms. Such symptoms are defined as:

1. unexplained weight loss of more than 10% in the six months before admission
2. unexplained fever with temperature above 38°C
3. night sweats.

Pruritus alone does not qualify for B classification, and a short febrile illness associated with a known infection does not qualify for B classification.

Staging of the disease is the single most important prognostic factor in Hodgkin's disease. B symptoms and bone marrow involvement are bad prognostic signs, while female patients and those less than 40 years old or with histological types 1 and 2 (section 18.3) have a better prognosis.

18.6 TREATMENT – CHOICE OF MODALITY

18.6.1 Radical treatment

In the large majority of cases, Hodgkin's disease is treated with curative intent. Radiotherapy alone is used for mantle, paraortic nodes and spleen for clinical stages IA, IIA, IIIA. Chemotherapy alone is used for IIIB and IV. Other stages (IB, IIB) should ideally be treated by chemotherapy and involved-fields radiotherapy. The method of treatment of stage IIIA (chemotherapy versus radiotherapy) is controversial.

18.6.2 Palliative treatment

At very advanced stages, only palliation can be offered to the patient. Chemotherapy and irradiation of symptomatic tumour masses can be very effective. Corticoids, blood transfusion, antibiotics and analgesics are of great importance.

18.7 RADIOTHERAPY TECHNIQUES

18.7.1 Radical mantle irradiation

This is performed for clinical stages IA-IIA. The target volumes are all the lymph nodes of the neck, axilla and mediastinum and a specially designed volume for the involved nodes. The prescribed dose is 36 Gy to areas of subclinical lymphatic involvement and 44 Gy to the nodes with gross clinical and/or radiological involvement. The technique involves an AP-PA mantle field with telecobalt.

- *Position.* Supine for both anterior and posterior mantle fields. If it is impossible to treat the posterior field with the head of the cobalt unit under the couch, the patient will have to be turned to the prone position for the posterior field. The hands should be on the hips with abduction of the elbows in a fixed and reproducible position. The head is fully extended to position the chin and the mastoid process on a nearly vertical line.
- *Localization.* Marks on the lower limit of both axillae.
- *Field margins* (Figures 18.1 and 18.2).
  The upper limit is a line drawn between the top of the extended chin and the mastoid process and occiput. The lower limit is

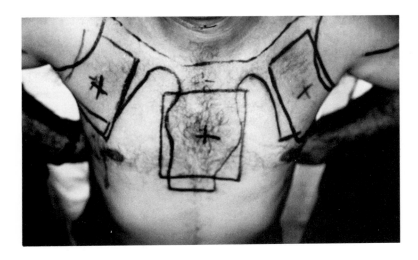

Figure 18.1 Radical mantle irradiation. Skin marks.

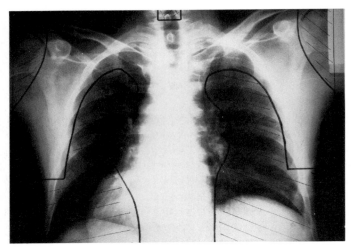

Figure 18.2 Radical mantle irradiation. Outline of the field limits on a radiograph.

between T10 and T11 for the mediastinum and the lower aspect of the axilla, usually at the level of the nipple. The lateral border is the external aspect of the axilla and the mediastinum with a margin of 2 cm.

- *Beam modification.* As the mantle field has a complex shape it is best to make an individualized adjusted block in cerobend with shielding of the humerus and lungs. A small block is used to shield the larynx and one may also shield the spine on the posterior field from the beginning or after 30 Gy. A small block is positioned on the spine at T10 if an inverted-Y field is anticipated to reduce the risk of field overlapping on the cord. A block is often positioned in the midline submental area for the last few fractions if the dose exceeds that of the greatest diameter of the mantle field.

- *Dose prescription.* The dose is prescribed midline on the central axis of the beam which usually lies in the upper part of the mediastinum. The total dose is 36 Gy in 20 fractions (180 cGy each). The dose must be calculated at all points of clinical interest for each session as the gaps are different from one point to another. The dose is calculated in the mediastinum (lower, mid- and upper mediastinum), neck nodes (subclavian, mid-jugular, mastoid) and mid-axilla. The dose to the spine and to the heart must also be calculated. When 36 Gy is given to any target volume, it is shielded from the mantle field until the end of the treatment. If there is a clinically detectable node(s), the pre-scribed dose will be 44 Gy. The boost dose of 8 Gy after 36 Gy can be given through reduced fields by fractions of 200 cGy each. A lateral field can be used for the mediastinum taking care not to overlap with the irradiation of the axilla and not exceeding 40 Gy on the spinal cord.

- *Special consideration.* When the thickness of the mediastinum is more than 20 cm (or even 18 cm), it is advisable whenever possible to use an X-ray beam of 10 MV or more. If customized cerobend blocks are not available, adjacent isocentric fields can be used to irradiate the neck, axilla and mediastinum separately.

18.7.2 Radical inverted-Y irradiation

This is performed alone in cases of infradiaphragmatic involvement or after the mantle field in stage III disease. The target volumes are all the lymph nodes of the paraortic, iliac and inguinal areas. The prescribed dose is 36 Gy to areas of subclinical lymphatic involvement and 44 Gy to nodes with gross lesions. The technique involves an asymmetric AP–PA inverted-Y field with telecobalt.

- *Position.* Supine for both anterior and posterior fields, but if it is impossible to treat the posterior field in this position, the patient will be turned to the prone position.
- *Localization.* Marks are positioned to delineate the lower border of the posterior field on the inguinal area. This will be the upper limit of the anterior inguinal field.
- *Field margins* (Figures 18.3 and 18.4). The upper limit of both fields is T12–L1. The lower limit of the posterior field is just above the femoral head along the pubic rim to encompass all the external iliac nodes. The lateral limits of the paraortic field is 1 cm lateral to the transverse processes. The lower limit of the anterior field is fixed clinically to encompass all the inguinal nodes. The inguinal region is irradiated only through this anterior Y field with a reduced field limited to this inguinal area. The upper border of this inguinal field is adjacent (with no overlap) to the inferior limit of the posterior Y field.

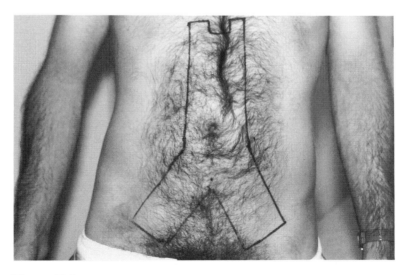

Figure 18.3 Radical inverted-Y irradiation. Skin marks.

- *Beam modification.* Customized blocks may be used to shield part of the abdomen and pelvis. A small block will shield the spinal cord at L1 if a mantle field has been irradiated previously.
- *Dose prescription.* The dose is prescribed midline on the central axis of the posterior Y field. The total dose is 36 Gy in 20 fractions. The dose must be calculated to the inguinal area at a depth of 2–3 cm according to the clinical situation, and, as this region is irradiated only through the anterior Y field, a boost dose is added to the small separate inguinal field to reach the total prescribed dose. If necessary, a boost dose of 8 Gy can be added through reduced field to any grossly involved nodes.
- *Special consideration.* When the interior–posterior diameter of the patient is more than 20 cm (or even 18 cm), it is recommended whenever possible to use X-ray beams of 10 MV or

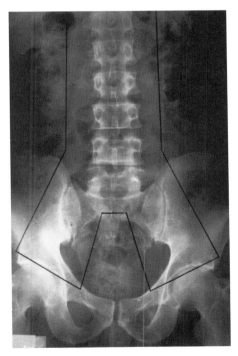

Figure 18.4 Radical inverted-Y irradiation. Outline of the field limits on a radiograph.

Table 18.2 Chemotherapy combinations for Hodgkin's disease

MOPP	ABVD
Mechlorethamine	Adriamycin
Vincristine	Bleomycin
Procarbazin	Vinblastin
Prednisone	Dicarbazine

more. Electrons are suitable to irradiate the inguinal area in association with cobalt or X-rays. The spleen can be included in the inverted-Y field, taking care to spare the lower half of the left kidney.

18.8 MORBIDITY

The acute reactions may include nausea, vomiting, dysphagia and diarrhoea. Temporary alopecia in the occipital area and xerostomia may occur depending on the upper limit of the mantle field. Haematopoietic depression is more likely after previous chemotherapy or with mantle and inverted-Y fields (total nodal irradiation).

Late effects may include radiation pneumonitis and pericarditis, chronic bowel changes and hypothyroidism. Careful treatment planning and field blocking, including so-called thin blocks in the cardiac region, will minimize late morbidity. Infertility in female patients can be avoided by ovarian transplantation when inverted-Y fields are necessary.

Late neoplasms may occur in up to 5% of cases treated by combinations of chemotherapy and large-field irradiation.

18.9 CHEMOTHERAPY

Chemotherapy is used for all stages with B symptoms, as well as stage IVA. Stage IIIA is preferably treated with chemotherapy followed by radiation consolidation therapy to involved sites.

Useful chemotherapy combinations for Hodgkin's disease are shown in Table 18.2. Toxicity from chemotherapy regimens prescribed for patients in developing countries may be unexpectedly higher and even fatal in tropical environments where nutritional deficiency and parasitic and bacterial infections are frequently seen in the population. Extreme caution in translating 'standard' chemotherapy schedules to other environments is indicated.

18.9.1 MOPP

Therapy is administered in 28-day cycles for two additional cycles beyond the attainment of a restaged complete remission, with a minimum of six cycles (months). Almost all patients who will achieve complete remission require eight months or less of treatment.

18.9.2 ABVD

This is an alternative regimen that appears to be as effective as MOPP but has much lower reported leukaemogenesis and infertility. Potential cardiac toxicity caused by adriamycin and potential pulmonary toxicity caused by bleomycin have occurred infrequently using this schedule and are of concern, especially when chemotherapy is combined with radiotherapy.

19

Non-Hodgkin's lymphoma

19.1 INCIDENCE AND RISK FACTORS

Non-Hodgkin's lymphoma (NHL) occurs at all ages (median 45 years), and the incidence increases with age. It is more frequent in developing countries. The cause is unknown.

19.1.1 Immunodeficiency states

Organ transplantation recipients, and those with congenital and acquired immunodeficiency syndromes (especially AIDS) and auto-immune disorders have an increased risk of non-Hodgkin's lymphoma.

19.1.2 Viruses

Members of the human type C retrovirus family have been implicated in the pathogenesis of at least one rare non-Hodgkin's lymphoma.

19.2 PRESENTATION AND NATURAL HISTORY

The tumour usually presents as a lump, mass or swelling. Untreated cases of NHL vary dramatically in terms of natural history, with prognoses ranging from days (e.g. Burkitt's lymphoma may have a tumour doubling time as brief as 24 hours) to decades.

In contrast to Hodgkin's disease, NHL presents with early bone marrow involvement (particularly the low-grade lymphomas), haematogenous and non-continuous spread, often involves extranodal

Table 19.1 Classification of malignant non-Hodgkin's lymphoma

Grade	Definition
Low	Diffuse, small lymphocytic
	Follicular, small cleaved
	Follicular, mixed, small cleaved and large cell
Intermediate	Follicular, large cleaved
	Diffuse, small cleaved
	Diffuse, mixed, small cleaved and large cell
	Diffuse, large cell (cleaved and non-cleaved ± sclerosis)
High	Diffuse, immunoblastic. Clear-cell (T-cell): pleomorphic
	Diffuse, lymphoblastic (convoluted and non-convoluted)
	Small, non-cleaved (follicular, rare, diffuse); Burkitt's

nodes, e.g. mesenteric and epitrochlear, and commonly originates in extranodal sites (especially the intermediate- and high-grade types).

Primary lymphoma of extranodal tissues, particularly gut, nasopharynx, bones and skin, occurs in up to a quarter of patients at presentation.

19.3 HISTOPATHOLOGY

The 'working formulation' (Table 19.1, Figure 19.1) divides lymphoma into low, intermediate and high grades reflecting their

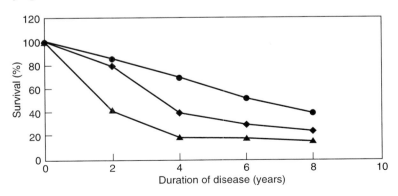

Figure 19.1 Survival curve for the working formulation (Table 19.1): (▲) high grade; (◆) intermediate grade; (●) low grade.

biological aggressiveness. The lower-grade lymphomas are characterized pathologically by the presence of small round lymphocytes and a nodular or follicular architecture of the lymphatic tissues, whereas the intermediate–high-grade lymphomas usually show larger cell size, prominent nucleoli, a high mitotic rate and disappearance of the normal follicular architecture of the nodes with a diffuse pattern of the lymphatic structures. It is usual to consider low-grade lymphomas as indolent or generally non-aggressive, while intermediate and high-grade lymphomas are considered as aggressive disease with a short natural history, if untreated.

19.4 INVESTIGATIONS

Investigations should include:

1. complete lymph node examination;
2. radiological studies:
   (a) chest radiograph: posterior–anterior lateral;
   (b) sonography of the abdomen and computed tomographic scan of thorax and abdomen if available;
3. full blood count;
4. liver function tests: serum LDH is a useful marker;
5. renal function studies to include urinalysis, serum creatinine, serum uric acid, serum electrolytes; and
6. bilateral bone marrow biopsy.

19.5 STAGING AND PROGNOSIS

The Ann Arbor classification (Table 18.1) is being adopted for the non-Hodgkin's lymphomas. The splenic and hepatic involvement in clinical staging as defined in the Ann Arbor classification is also used for non-Hodgkin's lymphomas. Prognosis and survival of the various forms are shown in Figure 19.1. Prognosis is worse in children and in elderly patients. Stage in itself is less important than in Hodgkin's disease. The cure rate has been improving as a result of more efficient chemotherapy regimens.

19.6 TREATMENT – CHOICE OF MODALITY

The choice of treatment modality will depend mainly on the histological type and also on the stage. Surgery may be indicated for

Table 19.2 Combination chemotherapy in non-Hodgkin's lymphoma

Acronym	Drugs
CVP	Cyclophosphamide Vincristine Prednisone
C-MOPP or COPP	Cyclophosphamide Vincristine Procarbazine Prednisone
CHOP	Cyclophosphamide Adriamycin Vincristine Prednisone

biopsy or splenectomy for palliation to remove a very large spleen or resection of the stomach, part of the small or large gut or the testis, etc. in primary extranodal NHL. For low-grade lymphoma, radiotherapy still plays an important role; for intermediate and high-grade lymphoma, chemotherapy is the cornerstone of treatment.

19.6.1 Therapy for low-grade lymphoma

1. Stage I/II disease is treated by radiotherapy of 40 Gy/20 fr/4 weeks to all sites of disease draining lymph nodes.
2. Stage III/IV
   (a) No treatment: however, therapy may be used in the presence of any systemic symptoms, rapid nodal growth or any complication of the disease such as anorexia, weight loss, obstructive symptoms or effusions.
   (b) Single-agent therapy with chlorambucil or cytoxan gives good responses that may develop slowly in indolent NHL.
   (c) Combination chemotherapy: if single agents fail, CVP or CHOP may be used (Table 19.2).
   (d) Palliative radiotherapy may be used to treat bulky disease and to relieve obstruction or pain.

19.6.2 Therapy for intermediate–high-grade lymphoma

Localized lesions (stage IA and IIA) can be managed by three cycles of CHOP followed by involved-field radiotherapy (30 Gy/10 fr/2 weeks). For stage II–IV disease, CHOP cures 30–35% of patients (Table 19.2).

Following treatment, masses should have resolved and serum LDH normalized. Maintenance therapy is not of value and is not recommended. LDH is a useful and inexpensive test to follow progress.

19.6.3 Therapy for lymphoblastic lymphoma

These patients should be managed as for acute lymphatic leukaemia.

20

Soft-tissue sarcoma

Soft-tissue sarcomas are a class of malignant tumours arising from mesenchymal structures and connective tissue cells.

20.1 INCIDENCE AND RISK FACTORS

Soft-tissue sarcomas are a rare group of tumours comprising nearly 1% of all adult malignant tumours. The annual age-adjusted incidence is 2 per 100 000. There is no sex bias. The commonest age of onset is 40–70 years. Previous irradiation is a predisposing factor.

20.2 PRESENTATION AND NATURAL HISTORY

The most common site of presentation is the extremities (60%), followed by the truncal area (30%), and the least common is the head and neck region.

The tumours appear as small, clinically innocuous lesions. Later, they grow, become symptomatic and often develop a hard consistency. Neurological or vascular symptoms may develop because of pressure effects.

20.3 HISTOPATHOLOGY

The main histological types are:

- alveolar soft-part sarcoma
- angiosarcoma

Table 20.1 Classification of soft-tissue sarcoma

Stage	Definition
TX	Primary tumour cannot be assessed
T0	No evidence of primary tumour
T1	Tumour $\leqslant$ 5 cm in greatest dimension
T2	Tumour $>$ 5 cm in greatest dimension

- epithelioid sarcoma
- extraskeletal chondrosarcoma
- extraskeletal osteosarcoma
- fibrosarcoma
- leiomyosarcoma
- liposarcoma
- malignant fibrous histiocytoma
- malignant haemangiopericytoma
- malignant mesenchymoma
- malignant Schwannoma
- rhabdomyosarcoma
- synovial sarcoma
- sarcoma NOS (not otherwise specified).

20.4 INVESTIGATIONS

Clinical examination is of prime importance. Biopsy is mandatory for diagnosis. Local extent is best determined by surgical exploration. If available, arteriography, computed tomography and increasingly, nuclear magnetic resonance imaging may be useful. A chest radiograph is mandatory but computed tomographic scans are more sensitive at detecting small metastatic lung nodules.

20.5 STAGING AND PROGNOSIS

The generally accepted primary classification for soft-tissue sarcomas (Russell *et al.*, 1977) is shown in Table 20.1. Stages I, II, and III are tumours that are histological grade 1, 2 and 3 respectively; substage A is used for tumours $\leqslant$ 5 cm in diameter and substage B for tumours $>$ 5 cm in diameter. Stage IV is defined as any grade of tumour with either invasion of major surrounding structures, such as vessels or nerves (IVA), or distant metastases (IVB).

20.5.1 Prognostic factors

Five-year survival is greater than 75% for well-differentiated tumours and less than 25% for poorly differentiated tumours. The site often influences the resectability and thus, local control and cure. The extent of local disease and of lymphatic or blood vessel invasion affect the prognosis.

Local recurrences after surgery alone are frequent and occur in 20–50% of cases. A first recurrence predisposes to further recurrences. It is highly probable that local recurrence is detrimental to survival.

20.6 TREATMENT – CHOICE OF MODALITY

20.6.1 Radical treatment

(a) Surgery

Wide adequate surgical resection is the commonest method of treatment. Excision of the sarcoma must be *en bloc* through normal tissues on all sides with at least a 3 cm margin on all sides of the biopsy scar. For radical excision, the tumour is removed with all tissue in the anatomical compartment occupied by the tumour.

Amputation of an involved limb is only indicated if the mass cannot be removed by wide excision, and operation would leave a useless limb without adequate neurovascular tissues or if the tumour is impossible to palliate by medical measures because of bleeding, pain or odour. Radical resection in an extremity can be achieved without amputation by replacing the bone with a prosthesis. This is generally not possible if there is significant vascular involvement and is not wise if major nerves must be sacrificed. This approach requires a significantly longer rehabilitation time and more effort than amputation.

Dissection of lymph nodes is generally not indicated unless the lesion is contiguous to major node-bearing areas or the nodes are involved. Solitary metastases should be removed, especially if these metastases appear late after excision of the primary tumour.

(b) Radiotherapy

Following wide excision, post-operative radiotherapy is performed to deliver approximately 65 Gy in $6\frac{1}{2}$ weeks using shrinking-field techniques.

(c) Chemotherapy

Chemotherapy for soft-tissue sarcoma in adults is not of value.

20.6.2 Palliative treatment

For palliation radiotherapy may give partial and sometimes complete response when large tumours are deemed unresectable. Short courses of irradiation can alleviate pain and prevent haemorrhage.

20.7 RADIOTHERAPY TECHNIQUES

20.7.1 Radical post-operative irradiation

This is performed 4–6 weeks after complete radical surgery to control subclinical residual disease in the tumour bed. The technique involves parallel opposed and shrinking fields with telecobalt for a tumour in the external part of the thigh. The target volume is the tumour bed with a safety margin of 6 cm around the tumour. The full length of the scar is part of the target volume. The prescribed dose is 60 Gy.

- *Position.* Prone with the foot in the vertical position.
- *Localization.* Radiopaque mark to localize the scar.
- *Field margins.*

    upper and lower limits: 6 cm below the gross tumour as identified on pre-operative radiographs or as delineated at the time of surgery (radiopaque clips)
    external limit: fall off (an average of 1.5 cm from the skin surface)
    internal limit: mid-shaft of femur

After 50 Gy, the fields are reduced to irradiate mainly the tumour site itself.

- *Beam modification*. Wedges are used to homogenize the dose in the target volume.
- *Dose prescription* (Figure 20.1). The total dose at the mid-axis is 60 Gy in 30 fractions over 6 weeks with field reduction after 50 Gy.
- *Special considerations*. Many different techniques can be used according to the size and mainly the site of the tumour. Blocks can be used to shield critical organs. Bolus can be placed over the scar to ensure full dosage on the skin surface. In the trunk and head and neck regions two- or three-wedge field techniques sometimes appear to be the best modality. In the limb, sparing of

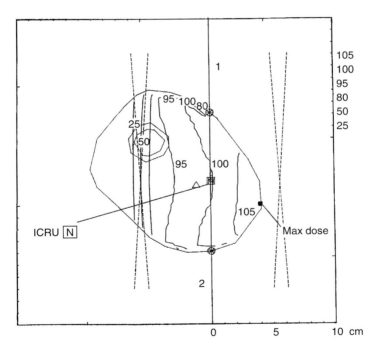

Figure 20.1 Radical post-operative irradiation. Isodose distribution for cobalt and SSD = 80 cm. [N] normalized on the 100% (ICRU) point; (■) maximum dose 110%. Loading: (1) anterior: 100 cGy/fr; (2) posterior: 100 cGy/fr.

a proportion of the circumference is essential in preventing distal oedema.

20.8 MORBIDITY

Acute side-effects mainly relate to skin reactions. After 6–18 months after treatment, fibrosis may develop. Severe fibrosis with bone necrosis should not be seen with a careful technique.

21

Central nervous system

The nervous system is composed of two parts, the central nervous system and the peripheral nervous system. The central nervous system is represented by the brain and spinal cord, while the peripheral nervous system consists of the spinal and cranial nerves. This chapter will deal exclusively with the central nervous system (CNS).

21.1 INCIDENCE AND RISK FACTORS

The incidence of CNS tumours varies with race (white > black), sex (men > women), and age. Although CNS tumours are the most common solid neoplasm of childhood, the incidence is about 17–20 in 100 000 between the ages of 65 and 80 years versus less than 2 in 100 000 for children less than 15 years old.

It has not been possible to identify an aetiological causative factor for human brain tumours. Recently, an increased incidence of brain lymphoma has been reported in patients with acquired immune deficiency syndrome. The association of some brain tumours with genetic factors (mostly autosomal dominant) has been recognized in neurofibromatosis (von Recklinghausen's disease and acoustic neuroma, optic nerve glioma and meningiomas), tuberous sclerosis (with astrocytomas), von Hippel–Lindau disease (with haemangioblastomas), Sturge–Weber syndrome (with astrocytomas), and familial polyposis (with meningioma and medulloblastoma). However, for the majority of brain tumours, such genetic disposition is lacking.

21.2 PRESENTATION AND NATURAL HISTORY

The symptomatology of cerebral tumours is usually gradual. Indeed, the hallmark of cerebral neoplasms is that they produce progressive neurological dysfunction that is dependent on the location, and rate of growth of the tumour and its surrounding oedema. Unlike metastatic disease, primary brain tumours are often solitary and very seldom produce sudden initial symptoms.

The neurological signs and symptoms caused by the tumours are related to two major mechanisms:

1. mass effect (either of the tumour or the tumour plus peritumoral oedema) causing increased intracranial or intraspinal pressure as the tumour mass expands within a fixed volume; and
2. infiltration of normal adjacent brain tissue by the tumour mass causing either destruction or irritation of neural tissue.

Increased intracranial pressure is frequently associated with most cerebral neoplasms and will usually produce headache, nausea/vomiting and drowsiness. Generalized convulsions or focal seizures are the presenting symptom in about 25% of patients with cerebral tumours. Personality change, hemiparesis, memory loss, speech impairment, cranial nerve deficit and sensory loss are also observed in 10–50% of cases.

The natural history of tumours of the CNS is relatively unique because even very malignant tumours rarely disseminate beyond the neuroaxis and they do not spread via lymphatic drainage. High-grade astrocytomas, medulloblastoma and dysgerminoma are among the few CNS tumours that infrequently metastasize through vascular channels with the bones and lung being the most frequent metastatic sites.

The large majority of CNS neoplasms have a characteristic growth pattern and tend to remain confined within the brain or spinal axis. Local spread usually occurs and will exert local pressure and infiltrative destruction. Certain tumours, such as meningiomas, may invade bone. Other tumours, because of their location, can cause displacement of vital structures, leading to life-threatening syndromes or severe neurological deficit. Metastatic seeding in the CNS space may occur in tumours such as medulloblastoma, ependymomas, high-grade infratentorial astrocytomas, and pineoblastomas.

21.3 HISTOPATHOLOGY

Several different terms have been applied to the same tumour types, resulting in confusing classifications and making treatment results somewhat difficult to interpret. Table 21.1 presents the WHO classification which is based on the presumed cell type of origin of the tumour (Zulch, 1979). The distinction between malignant and benign tumours is only made on histopathological grounds. A 'benign' tumour may produce devastating neurological deficits in a relatively short time because of its location, whereas a histologically malignant lesion may not produce any symptoms for several months or years. Whenever indicated, the histopathological degree of differentiation should be clearly stated because of its important prognostic implications in some of the malignant neoplasms.

Table 21.1 Pathological classification of central nervous system cancers

Cell type or origin	Tumour type
Neuroglial cells	Astrocytomas (grades I–IV)
	Oligodendrogliomas
	Ependymomas
Neuronal cells and primitive	Medulloblastomas
biopotential precursors	Neuroblastomas
	Ganglioneuroma and ganglioglioma
Mesodermal tissues	Meningiomas
	Sarcomas
Spine and nerve roots	Schwannomas
	Neurofibromas
Lymphoreticular system	Lymphomas (microglioma)
	Plasmacytoma
	Leukaemias
Pineal region	Germinomas (pinealoma)
Germ-cell origin	Teratomas
	Choriocarcinoma
	Embryonal carcinoma
Pineal parenchyma	Pineocytoma
	Pineoblastoma
Choroid plexus	Choroid plexus papilloma
Maldevelopmental origin	Craniopharyngioma
	Teratoma
Pituitary gland	
Blood vessels	Haemangioblastoma
	Arteriovenous malformations
Metastatic tumours	

21.4 INVESTIGATIONS

The use of computed tomography (CT) and more recently of magnetic resonance imaging (MRI) has revolutionized the investigation of patients with CNS tumours. A CT scan is a non-invasive procedure that usually enables anatomical localization of the lesion and differentiation between tumour and oedema. The use of iodine contrast is very helpful in providing information about tumour extension by enhancing areas in where the blood–brain barrier has been disrupted. A new paramagnetic contrast agent (gadolinium–DTPA), which crosses leaky tumour vessels, is now in clinical use and has proven to be useful in determining tumour extension.

Radionuclide scanning may be useful if neither CT nor MRI is available. Technetium is the isotope commonly used. Brain scintigraphy has poor resolution.

Cerebral angiography was frequently used prior to the advent of CT scanning. It was usually done pre-operatively to determine the relationship between the tumour and major vessels. Its major indication now is for vascular lesions such as arteriovenous malformations and aneurysms.

Myelography is useful to demonstrate neuroaxis seeding and spinal cord tumours. It plays an important role in establishing the precise level of the lesion (primary or metastatic) prior to radiotherapy planning. CT scan and MRI have now largely replaced myelography, particularly in extramedullary lesions.

21.5 STAGING AND PROGNOSIS

In its 1987 edition, the UICC produced a staging system which applies to all brain tumours (Tables 21.2 and 21.3). This classification is divided according to whether the tumour is supratentorial or infratentorial and is based on physical examination findings and imaging studies performed to assess tumour extension. It has not been widely used and this may in part be due to the heterogeneity and biological behaviour of brain neoplasms with pathologically similar neoplasms having entirely different clinical courses simply based on the anatomical structures involved. The American Joint Committee on Cancer has also published a similar staging system based on grade, size and location of the tumour, and the presence of metastatic disease, including neuroaxis seeding. Like the UICC

Table 21.2 Classification of brain tumours

Stage	Definition
T	*Primary tumour*
TX	Primary tumour cannot be assessed
T0	No evidence of primary tumour
Supratentorial tumours	
T1	Tumour $\leq$ 5 cm in greatest diameter, limited to one side
T2	Tumour $>$ 5 cm in greatest diameter, limited to one side
T3	Tumour invades or encroaches on the ventricular system
T4	Tumour crosses the midline of the brain, invades the opposite hemisphere or invades infratentorially
Infratentorial tumours	
T1	Tumour $\leq$ 3 cm in greatest diameter, limited to one side
T2	Tumour $>$ 3 cm in greatest diameter, limited to one side
T3	Tumour invades or encroaches on the ventricular system
T4	Tumour crosses the midline of the brain, invades the opposite hemisphere or invades supratentorially
M	*Distant metastasis*
MX	Presence of distant metastasis cannot be assessed
M0	No distant metastasis
M1	Distant metastasis
G	*Histopathological grading*
GX	Grade cannot be assessed
G1	Well differentiated
G2	Moderately differentiated
G3	Poorly differentiated
G4	Undifferentiated

classification, its use has also been very limited. A staging system for medulloblastoma based on radiographic and operative evaluation of tumour extent and subarachnoid metastasis has been proposed by Chang.

A number of variables of prognostic significance have been established for brain neoplasms. Age appears to be the most important prognostic factor, with younger patients faring better than older ones. Histological grading also correlates strongly with survival. Other factors known to be of prognostic value include the performance status of the patients, the degree of surgical resection,

Table 21.3 Stage grouping

Stage	TNM classification		
IA	G1	T1	M0
1B	G1	T2, T3	M0
IIA	G2	T1	M0
IIB	G2	T2, T3	M0
IIIA	G3	T1	M0
IIIB	G3	T2, T3	M0
IV	G1	T4	M0
	G2	T4	M0
	G3	T4	M0
	G4	Any T	M0
	Any G	Any T	M1

the presence of necrosis, tumour location, and duration of symptoms. Table 21.4 shows the survival rates after various treatments.

21.6 RADIOTHERAPY TECHNIQUES

21.6.1 Partial brain irradiation

This is used when treating patients with curative intent. The aim of such a technique is to give a high and homogeneous dose in the target volume and to spare as much as possible the rest of the brain structures. It may involve irradiation alone of a small primary lesion or, as in the technique described here, post-operative irradiation after complete gross resection of a low-grade astrocytoma.

The target volume is the primary tumour with a safety margin of 2 cm all around. A CT scan and the operative report and close collaboration with the neurosurgery team are essential for an accurate definition of the target volume and critical organs. The prescribed dose is 45 Gy. The technique is a four-field box technique with telecobalt.

- *Position.* Supine with the head extended in such a way that the vertical AP–PA beam does not pass through the eyes. This may sometimes require that the neck be strongly flexed with the chin on the sternal notch. An individual mask is useful to provide good and reproducible positioning.
- *Localization.* This is done according to the known anatomical situation of the target volume and clinical landmarks of the

Table 21.4 Treatment results for intracranial tumours

Tumour	Five-year survival
Astrocytoma	
Grade I	Surgery alone (partial resection): 25%
	Surgery + radiotherapy: 58%
Grade II	Surgery alone (partial resection): 0%
	Surgery + radiotherapy: 25%
Grade III	< 10% (median survival 25–30 months)
Grade IV	0% (median survival 6–8 months)
	Radiotherapy + BCNU, median survival 8 months
Oligodendroglioma	Surgery alone: 23–82%
	Surgery + radiotherapy: 53–100%
Ependymoma	Surgery alone: 15–25%
Low grade	Radiotherapy: 75%
High grade	Radiotherapy: 10–50%
Medulloblastoma	Overall: 50%
	Good risk: 65–70%
	Poor risk: 25–30%
Pineal tumours	Germinoma: 70–5%
	Parenchymal cell 20–25%
Lymphomas	< 10%
Craniopharyngiomas	Overall: 80–100%
	Children: 90–100%
	Adults: 60–90%

different brain and base-of-skull structures. A CT scan in the position of treatment with the field delineated is the best way to ensure proper positioning of the beam.

- *Field margins* (Figures 21.1 and 21.2). These take into account a 2 cm safety margin around the clinical target volume in three dimensions. Base-of-skull, midline of the brain, mid-brain and cerebellum are useful landmarks for good delineation of these field margins. The field sizes are usually 7–10 cm × 7–10 cm.
- *Dose prescription* (Figures 21.3 and 21.4). The total dose is 45 Gy in 25 fractions. The dose per fraction is 180 cGy.
- *Special considerations.* When available an X-ray beam of 8 MV or more will give better dose distribution. Lead blocks can be added to protect a specific critical organ in the brain. The dose

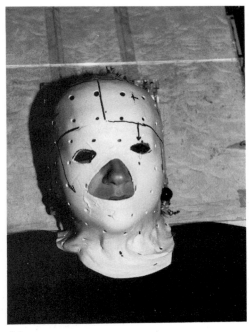

(a)

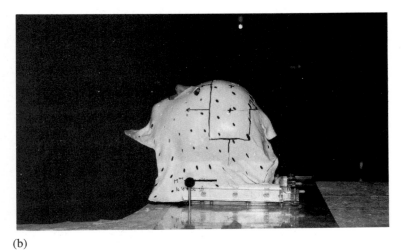

(b)

Figure 21.1 Partial brain irradiation. Skin marks: (a) anterior field; (b) lateral field.

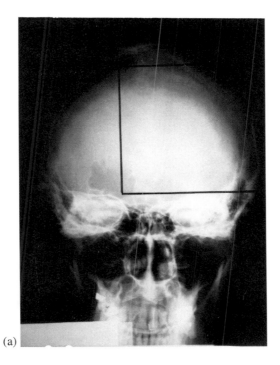

(a)

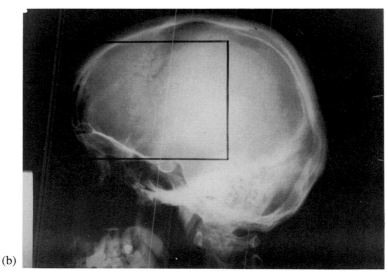

(b)

Figure 21.2 Partial brain irradiation. Outline of the field limits on a radiograph: (a) anterior field; (b) lateral field.

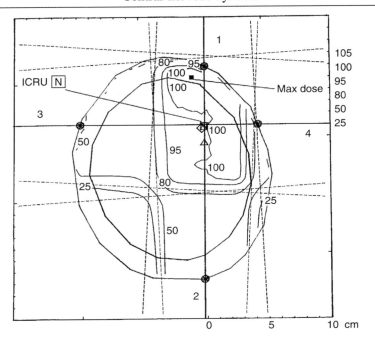

Figure 21.3 Partial brain irradiation. Isodose distribution for cobalt and SSD = 80 cm. N normalized on the 100% (ICRU) point; (■) maximum dose 103%. Loading: (1) anterior: 55 cGy/fr; (2) posterior: 55 cGy/fr; (3) right lateral: 45 cGy/fr; (4) left lateral; 45 cGy/fr.

per fraction can be modified up to 200 cGy in 5 fractions per week. The beam loading may vary according to the location of the tumour and the need for low dose in a specific brain area.

21.6.2 Pituitary irradiation

Such irradiation may be proposed for an incompletely resected adenoma to control residual growth. The target volume is the sella turcica, with safety margins according to the location of the adenoma with either intra- or suprasellar extension or invasion of the cavernous sinus laterally. A CT scan and MRI are essential for a good definition of the tumour volume. The prescribed dose is 50.40 Gy with daily fractions of 180 cGy. The technique is a three-field technique with wedges and telecobalt.

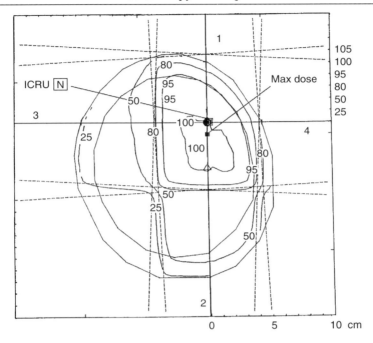

Figure 21.4 Partial brain irradiation. Isodose distribution for 18 MV and SAD. $\boxed{N}$ normalized on the 100% (ICRU) point; (■) maximum dose 100%. Loading: (1) anterior: 55 cGy/fr; (2) posterior: 55 cGy/fr; (2) posterior: 55 cGy/fr; (3) right lateral: 45 cGy/fr; (4) left lateral; 45 cGy/fr.

- *Position.* Supine with the patient's neck flexed so that the anterior field will miss the eyes.
- *Localization.* It is usually easy to locate the centre of the sella turcica and its bony structures.
- *Field margins* (Figure 21.5). The field size is usually 5–7 cm × 5–7 cm depending on the tumour dimensions:

  lower limit: at the lower part of the sphenoidal sinus
  anterior, upper, lateral limits: usually 2 cm around the sella turcica if there is no extrasellar extension

- *Dose prescription* (Figure 21.6). The total dose is 50.40 Gy in 28 fractions of 180 cGy each, 5 fractions per week.

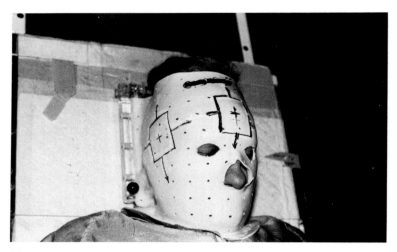

Figure 21.5 Radical irradiation of the pituitary. Skin marks for anterior and lateral fields.

21.6.3 Whole-brain irradiation

This technique is used for metastatic brain disease, with palliative intent. The target volume is the whole brain and meninges. The prescribed dose is 30 Gy in 10 fractions. The technique involves two parallel opposed lateral fields with telecobalt.

- *Position.* Supine.
- *Localization.* The base of skull is the main landmark easily seen on the control film or fluoroscopic control. The external contours of the orbits may be delineated and a radiopaque marker may be used to outline the external auditory canal.
- *Field margins* (Figures 21.7 and 21.8).

  lower limit: 1 cm below the base of the skull taking care to encompass the temporal lobes, fully
  anterior, posterior, upper limits: the anatomical edges of the skull

- *Dose prescription.* Total dose is 30 Gy in 10 fractions over 2 weeks, i.e. an accelerated schedule of 5 fractions per week, 300 cGy per fraction.

• *Special considerations.* The lower limit may be a straight line but a block can be positioned on the orbit to shape the field to the base of skull.

21.6.4 Craniospinal irradiation

Certain neoplasms have a tendency for metastatic spread to spinal cord. Thus patients with such tumours, in addition to cranial irradiation, should also have the spinal axis electively treated. Irradiation of the entire subarachnoid space is technically demanding and requires the full participation of several members of a radiation oncology department, including physics staff and mould room personnel, if a mould room is available.

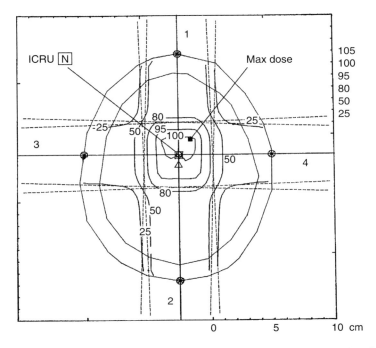

Figure 21.6 Radical irradiation of the pituitary. Isodose distribution for cobalt and SSD = 80 cm. $\boxed{N}$ normalized on the 100% (ICRU) point; ($\blacksquare$) maximum dose 101%. Loading: (1) anterior: 40 cGy/fr; (2) posterior: 40 cGy/fr; (3) right lateral: 50 cGy/fr; (4) left lateral; 50 cGy/fr.

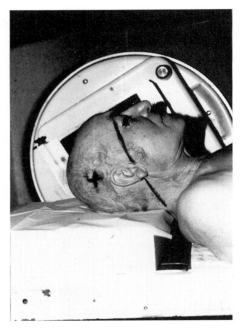

Figure 21.7 Whole-brain irradiation. Skin marks.

The goal of craniospinal irradiation is to cover the treatment volume as uniformly as possible, and usually three or four fields are required in order to achieve this target. Proper set-up and careful calculations are necessary. Particular attention must be observed at the junctional zones to avoid overdosage or underdosage and to ensure accurate delivery of the irradiation.

Several craniospinal techniques have been described and are in clinical use. Because of its simplicity and easy reproducibility, we suggest use of the technique described by Van Dyke *et al*. In the technique, a telecobalt unit with a source-to-surface distance of 80 cm is used for all fields. The patient is treated in the prone position and adequate immobilization devices must be available to ensure daily treatment reproducibility.

The head is treated by parallel opposed lateral fields which will include the whole brain and the cervical spine to C3–C4. The face, eyes and anterior part of the neck are shielded with individually cut-out 5 cm thick lead blocks placed laterally at a distance of ± 30 cm

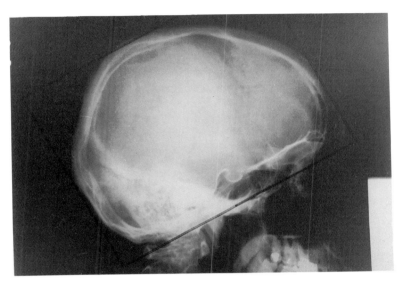

Figure 21.8 Whole-brain irradiation. Outline of the field limits on a radiograph.

from the face. The head fields are rotated $10.5°$ such that the inferior border of these fields follows the line of divergence of the upper spine field. Partial shielding of the cervical vertebral body should be avoided to prevent deformity during bone growth.

The spinal cord is treated by one or two direct posterior fields at a source-to-surface distance of 80 cm. For the upper spine field, the collimator setting is kept constant at a length of 30 cm. This will keep the line of divergence at the edge of the field at a constant angle with respect to the central radiograph. Consequently, the angle of rotation of the lateral fields ($10.5°$) can be kept constant for all patients. In the unusual case that the total length of the spine field is less than 30 cm, a shielding block is placed at the inferior border of the beam to give the desired length (the collimator aperture remains at 30 cm). For the majority of patients, however, a second posterior spine field needs to be added, as the total length of the spine is rarely less than 30 cm. This second spine field will not have a predetermined collimator setting and its length will be dependent on the total spine length. A gap is left between the two spine fields, with the length of the gap depending, of course, on the depth at which the fields are to be matched and the length of each of the spine fields.

To avoid under- or overdosage at the field junctions, both junctions are moved 5–10 mm inferiorly after each 8–10 Gy has been delivered. It is important to realize that the lower border of the inferior spine field is kept the same (usually the inferior border of the second sacral segment) and, therefore, this field needs to be decreased by the same length for each move. Since the head fields are also moved inferiorly, enough margin must be cleared superiorly so that no part of the intracranial contents is improperly shielded.

21.6.5 Palliative treatment

Metastatic disease to the brain and spinal cord constitutes the most common reason for application of palliative treatment within the central nervous system. Resection of solitary brain lesions may be considered in patients with a good performance status, no other evident metastatic lesions, controlled primary lesion and anatomically accessible disease in the brain. Post-operative irradiation is generally recommended following resection. Treatment recommendations for solitary metastases occurring in patients not fitting the criteria for resection or in the case of multiple intracranial lesions are dependent on clinical presentation. Patients with good to excellent functional status, control of the primary tumour, age less than 60 years and limited extent of metastatic disease may be candidates for high-dose localized irradiation. In patients with multiple or more advanced metastatic disease, short courses of radiation delivered as either 20 Gy in 5 fractions or 30 Gy in 10 fractions to the whole brain are recommended. The optimal dose schedule for treatment of spinal cord metastases has not been determined; however, dose fractionation similar to that used for brain metastases is commonly applied.

21.7 SPECIFIC INTRACRANIAL TUMOUR TYPES

21.7.1 Astrocytomas

Astrocytomas are usually classified as low grade or high grade depending on their histopathological appearance. The low-grade astrocytomas, sometimes referred as 'benign' astrocytomas, have a slower growth pattern than the high-grade astrocytomas, also known as 'malignant' astrocytomas.

The classification of these tumours as benign and malignant is somewhat misleading because, with the exception of a few low-grade tumours that can be completely resected, even grade I and II tumours behave in a malignant fashion and can be lethal.

(a) Low-grade astrocytomas

Low-grade astrocytomas include grade I and II tumours. They represent about 8% of primary intracranial neoplasms and up to 18% of all astrocytomas. These tumours are slow-growing and symptoms may antedate the discovery of the tumours by years.

(b) High-grade astrocytomas

Grade III and IV astrocytomas, also known as malignant astro-cytomas and glioblastoma multiforme, are the most common brain tumour in adults. The age of peak incidence is 45–55 years. These tumours are rapidly growing with a uniformly fatal prognosis.

21.7.2 Oligodendrogliomas

Oligodendrogliomas constitute about 5% of primary intracranial gliomas. Classically, they are slow-growing and have a long natural history with a median survival of over five years following the onset of symptoms. The frontal lobes are the most frequently involved region and abnormal calcifications may be seen on skull radio-graphs. The peak incidence is in persons between 30 and 50 years old.

The role of post-operative radiotherapy in these gliomas is not clear. Nevertheless, the limited available data suggest that post-operative radiotherapy improves five-year survival of these patients. Five-year survival rates following surgery alone range from 23% to 82%, and with irradiation range from 53% to 100%.

21.7.3 Ependymoma

Ependymomas occur in all age groups, although they are more frequent in children and young adults. They constitute 5–8% of intracranial gliomas. They arise from the lining cells of the ventricles, with the majority occurring below the tentorium, in the midline of the fourth ventricle. About 30% will grow through the foramen magnum, extending into the cervical spine. The majority of ependymomas cannot be completely resected because of their location and pattern of growth. Grading and location are the most important factors in prognosis, with high-grade supratentorial tumours having the worst survival. Some 60% of intracranial ependymomas are infratentorial and 40% are supratentorial. The five-year survival rates with surgery alone range from 15% to 25%. The addition of post-operative radiotherapy has improved survival in children and adults with this disease and is now accepted as standard therapy.

21.7.4 Medulloblastoma

Medulloblastoma is a primitive tumour of neuroextodermal origin occurring in the midline of the cerebellum. It accounts for 15–20% of intracranial childhood tumours. In older age groups, a 'sarcomatous' variant, which has similar biological behaviour, may occur laterally in the cerebellum and should be treated in the same way.

Medulloblastomas are known for their high tendency to recur locally and to metastasize. At presentation up to 20–30% of patients will have positive cytology or myelographic evidence of spinal metastasis. Extraneural metastasis, although occurring in less than 5% of cases, is more frequently seen in medulloblastoma than in any other CNS tumour. Most metastasis are to bone, bone marrow, lymph nodes or lung.

Radiotherapy plays a major role in the management of this disease. Before the use of radiation therapy, the disease tended to run an almost always fatal course with few patients surviving more than five years. Prior to 1970, the five-year survival rate was about 35%. Recently, following modern craniospinal irradiation, five-year survival rates of 50–60% or higher have been reported. Factors related to prognosis include age (children less than two years old have poorer disease control) and disease extension. The majority of recurrences appear within two or three years after treatment and the posterior fossa is the most common site of initial tumour recurrence.

21.7.5 Meningioma

Meningiomas are tumours that arise from the arachnoidal cells in the meninges. The large majority are histologically benign, with low proliferative capacity and limited invasiveness, although, less commonly, anaplastic meningiomas may occur. Their peak incidence is in the fourth and fifth decades and they are twice as common in women. Meningiomas may arise wherever arachnoidal cells are present but are most frequently located along the sagittal sinus and cerebral convexity. Benign meningioma constitutes 15% of adult CNS tumours.

Meningiomas are well circumscribed and generally do not invade the underlying brain parenchyma. Surgery is the mainstay of treatment, although complete resection is not always possible because these tumours may be extremely vascular or may surround important structures.

The role of radiotherapy is still somewhat controversial. While some authors recommend irradiation of all incompletely resected tumours, some others contend that recurrent meningiomas may be controlled by irradiation and that this treatment modality should therefore be reserved for recurring disease. For patients undergoing complete resection, the recurrence rate is less than 5%. In contrast, subtotal removal carries a recurrence rate of 50–75%. For those patients who receive post-operative irradiation following subtotal resection, the recurrence drops to less than 30%.

21.7.6 Pineal region tumours

Tumours of the pineal and suprasellar regions are rare (less than 1% of all CNS tumours; 3–5% of CNS childhood tumours), although in countries such as Japan they account for 5–8% of brain tumours. The peak incidence is in the first two decades of life. Germinomas (also referred to as pinealomas, dysgerminomas or atypical teratomas) are the most common tumours, accounting for more than 50% of cases. Gliomas account for 25% of pineal tumours and tumours of pineal parenchymal origin represent about 15%. Prognosis is dependent on histology, size of tumour, and tumour extension. Five-year survival rates following radiation therapy vary from 50% to 80%. Radiotherapy is clearly indicated in most pineal tumours.

21.7.7 Lymphomas

Primary intracranial lymphomas account for < 1% of all intracranial tumours. The peak incidence is in the fifth and sixth decades. They usually arise in the supratentorial region, although they may also occur in the cerebellum and brain stem. During the last few years, a substantial increase in incidence has been reported in immunosuppressed patients, especially in patients with acquired immune deficiency syndrome. Lesions are multifocal in 5–40% of the cases.

Prognosis is rather poor, with a one-year survival rate of 66%, a two-year survival rate of 43%, and five-year survival rate of less than 10%. The vast majority of lymphomas recur at the primary site.

21.7.8 Pituitary tumours

Tumours in the pituitary region constitute 6–10% of intracranial neoplasms. The majority arise from the adenohypophysis and classically were classified as chromophobe adenomas (85% of all cases), acidophil adenomas, and basophil adenomas. Some of the endocrine abnormalities associated with pituitary adenomas include sexual impotence in the male and amenorrhoea and galactorrhoea in the female in prolactin-secreting tumours, gigantism or acromegaly in hypersecretion of growth hormone, and Cushing's disease with ACTH hypersecretion. Local disease extension, suprasellar or extra-sellar, determines symptomatology. Bi-temporal hemianopia is the chief visual deficit and headache occurs in 20% of cases.

21.7.9 Craniopharyngiomas

Craniopharyngioma is a tumour that originates from the remnants of Rathke's pouch in the region of the pituitary stalk. They occur primarily in children and about 80% will show some degree of calcification. They can cause symptoms by compressing the optic chiasm or tracts, depressing pituitary or hypothalamic functions, increasing the intracranial pressure or all of these. Tumours become symptomatic usually after they reach a diameter of about 3 cm. Radiotherapy is effective in these tumours and should be given to patients with less than total resection.

21.8 SPINAL CORD TUMOURS

Intraspinal neoplasms account for about 10% of all primary CNS tumours. These tumours can be extremely disabling and prompt recognition and treatment is very important to relieve the morbidity. The majority of primary spinal tumours are intradural. The commonest intradural tumours are neurilemmomas (Schwannoma), meningiomas, astrocytomas and ependymomas. Neurilemmomas and meningiomas are frequently extramedullary, while the gliomas tend to be intramedullary. The clinical manifestations are caused by compression of the spinal cord or cauda equina, leading to weakness and sensory abnormalities. Pain, which can be quite intense, may develop because of external compression and infiltration of spinal cord roots. Radiotherapy is recommended for incompletely resected tumours.

21.9 MORBIDITY

Acute toxicity is mainly related to the skin with alopecia associated with brain irradiation. Radiation to the brain can also result in headache, nausea, lethargy (often described as a 'somnolence syndrome' in the post-radiation period) and otitis media. Sequelae associated with spinal radiation depend on location of the treatment field and adjacent normal structures, including the mucosal surfaces of the oesophagus and the bowel. Late necrosis of the brain is a risk in long-term survivors. With so few surviving with the diagnosis of malignant glioma, therapeutic controversy remains with respect to selection of dosage.

22

Retinoblastoma

Retinoblastoma is a malignant tumour arising from the embryonic retina. It is the most common intra-ocular tumour of childhood and may originate from single or multiple foci in one or both eyes. It is highly curable in early stages without significant loss of vision. It has autosomal dominant inheritance and a tendency for bilaterality.

22.1 INCIDENCE AND RISK FACTORS

Retinoblastoma is a relatively rare tumour and constitutes about 3–5% of all childhood malignancies. The usual time of occurrence is in childhood but the tumour is also occasionally seen at birth. About 80% of cases are diagnosed before the age of 3–4 years. Bilateral cases are diagnosed earlier than unilateral cases. The ratio of unilateral to bilateral cases in any large series may reflect the deficiencies in referral to specialized centres.

The aetiology of retinoblastoma is not known, but hereditary and non-hereditary forms are known to exist. Approximately 90% of newly diagnosed cases are sporadic, without any family history of retinoblastoma. In 20–25% of cases of inherited retinoblastoma, a characteristic deletion is seen in the q14 band of chromosome 13. In non-germinal forms, this deletion is seen only in tumour cells, whereas in the inherited variety, deletion is seen in all the cells of the body.

Retinoblastoma is characterized by rapid growth and has been said to have a spontaneous regression rate of 1%. Patients with heritable retinoblastoma have a substantial risk of developing a second malignant tumour. The second tumours are predominantly sarcomas with osteosarcoma being the most common.

22.2 PRESENTATION AND NATURAL HISTORY

The most common sign is leucokoria (a white reflex of the eye) (56%), first identified by parents. Leucokoria is first seen when the tumour is fairly large. The next most common presenting sign is strabismus (20%), which occurs when tumour arises in the macula. Other presenting findings in advanced stages are painful eye with glaucoma (7%), visual disturbance (5%), orbital cellulitis, unilateral dilatation of the pupil, heterochromia, hyphaema and nystagmus.

22.3 HISTOPATHOLOGY

Most tumour cells are undifferentiated small cells with hyper-chromatic nuclei of various sizes and scanty cytoplasm with plenty of mitotic figures. The tumour has a tendency to outgrow its blood supply, with resulting necrosis. Retinoblastoma can be endophytic if the tumour grows mainly from the inner surface of the retina toward the vitreous humour or exophytic where the tumours grow from the outer layers of retina towards the subretinal space. Retinal detach-ment is common with large tumours. Vitreous seeding may also occur.

Retinoblastoma spreads by direct extension into the orbit along scleral draining vessels, by invasion of the optic nerve, by the haematogenous route or by lymphatic extension.

22.4 INVESTIGATIONS

The diagnosis of retinoblastoma is usually established clinically by an experienced ophthalmologist by ophthalmoscopic examination of the eye. Pupillary dilatation and examination under anaesthesia are essential to evaluate the retina fully. Intra-ocular calcification and the formation of vitreous seeds are almost pathognomic of a retinoblastoma. Calcium can be seen with the ophthalmoscope in over 50% of the lesions. If the tumour is not well visualized on fundoscopic examination, radiophosphate-32 localization of the tumour and radiograph studies may assist diagnosis. Roentgeno-graphic studies of the skull may demonstrate the presence of intra-ocular calcification and/or the involvement of the orbit by tumour.

Table 22.1 Reese staging of retinoblastoma: St Bartholomew's modification

Stage	Definition
I	Single or multiple tumours less than 4 disc diameters at or behind the equator (one disc diameter = 1.5 mm)
IIA	Solitary lesion 4–10 disc diameters at or behind the equator
IIB	Solitary lesion larger than 10 disc diameters at or behind the equator
III	Lesions anterior to the equator
IVA	Multiple tumours, some larger than 10 disc diameters
IVB	Any lesion extending anteriorly beyond the limit of ophthalmology
VA	Massive neoplasms
VB	Vitreous seedings
VI	Residual orbital disease or optic nerve infiltration

Ultrasonography is another helpful non-invasive procedure. Computed tomography is useful in demonstrating intra-ocular extent as well as possible extra-ocular extension.

22.5 STAGING AND PROGNOSIS

Reliable and quick diagnosis and evaluation are important since retinoblastoma has a rapid growth rate. Early diagnosis is extremely important because the prognosis for visual acuity is related to tumour size at the initiation of treatment. Table 22.1 shows an accepted staging scheme.

The cure rate among patients with unilateral retinoblastoma confined to the globe is over 90%. However, survival of patients with bilateral retinoblastoma is extremely poor because of a high incidence of secondary malignancy. Successful treatment is measured in terms of eradication of disease with preservation of useful vision.

22.6 TREATMENT – CHOICE OF MODALITY

Eighty per cent of children with retinoblastoma can expect cure with reasonable sight with modern methods of radiotherapy. Enucleation is sparingly undertaken in modern practice and the indications for enucleation are limited to massive tumours and those involving or overlying the disc when unilateral and when the chance of useful vision in that eye is extremely low. Ever since preservation of vision became a major objective of treatment, radiotherapy has assumed an increasingly important role in this tumour.

For small tumours less than 3 mm in diameter which are quite posteriorly situated laser coagulation or photocoagulation can be employed to destroy unilateral or bilateral tumours. For the more anterior lesions, this method is difficult to employ and cryotherapy is used in such situations.

Larger tumours (3–10 mm) are treated with telecobalt plaques or iodine-125 plaques. The dose is calculated for the apex of the tumour to deliver 40 Gy. The operation is performed jointly by the ophthalmologist and radiotherapist. A plaque of appropriate size is sutured to the base of the growth after proper exposure and ophthalmoscopic control. The results of this therapy are excellent. However, it is not easily used in cases of a lesion near the macula and optic disc.

When the lesion is more than 10–12 mm in diameter or when there are multiple tumours, in the presence of vitreous seeding or when the tumours are situated near macula or disc, external beam radiation is preferred. Since there is a high incidence of relapse, whole-eye irradiation using anterior and lateral fields or a single anterior field is preferred, accepting the ultimate morbidity of cataract and loss of vision in centres where less sophisticated equipment is available. In centres where conformational therapy can be achieved, the recently evolved Utrecht technique may be used to apply beam-directed radiation to the whole retina and vitreous humour. The dose used is 35 Gy in 15 fractions as this is an extremely sensitive tumour.

Response to radiotherapy will be obvious within 4–6 weeks after completion of therapy. If a small residual tumour is present after treatment, it can be safely treated with local implants or coagulation methods. The major complications are cataract, usually two years later, which can be easily treated with lens aspiration and correction of vision, xerophthalmia and growth retardation of the orbit.

Invasion of the choroid and the presence of tumours in the cut end of the optic nerve predispose enucleated cases to a very high chance of distant metastases whereas local recurrence can be reduced by post-operative radiotherapy. Post-operative X-ray irradiation to the orbit is given up to 35 Gy in 15 fractions with an anterior field or a pair of anterior and lateral wedged fields.

The role of chemotherapy for retinoblastoma remains undefined. Shrinkage of ocular tumours has been demonstrated in patients treated prior to enucleation with cyclophosphamide, doxorubicin and vincristine, but no clear survival advantage over enucleation alone was seen by their adjuvant use. Because effective local control and survival is achieved in 90% of patients given local treatment (surgery or radiotherapy), chemotherapy is restricted to patients with extra-ocular disease. Even in extra-ocular retino-blastoma, the responses are unsatisfactory and are of short duration. Combination chemotherapy using vincristine, adriamycin and en-doxan, adriamycin and *cis*-platin, VM-26 has also achieved only partial responses.

23

Wilms' tumour (nephroblastoma)

Wilms' tumour is a malignant embryonal tumour arising from the kidney. It is also known as renal embryoma or nephroblastoma. The mortality rate was more than 80% during the early years of the 20th century. However, with advances in surgery, radiation therapy and chemotherapy, five-year survival rates have now increased to more than 80%.

23.1 INCIDENCE AND RISK FACTORS

The incidence of Wilms' tumour is 7.8 per million population in those aged 1–14 years. Thus approximately one child in 100 000 develops a Wilms' tumour. There is relatively little geographic variation in incidence. It constitutes about 6–7% of all childhood tumours.

The neoplasm is most common in young children: 77% occur in children less than five years old and 90% occur in those less than seven years old. The median age is $3\frac{1}{2}$ years. Male and female children are affected equally. It occurs in both hereditary and non-hereditary forms.

Wilms' tumour shows a strong association with certain congenital anomalies: aniridia, hemihypertrophy, genito-urinary malformations especially in boys, and Beckwith–Weidemann syndrome. Parental prenatal exposure to occupational toxins, specifically lead and hydrocarbons, has been implicated as causative but this has not been proved.

23.2 PRESENTATION AND NATURAL HISTORY

Most patients with Wilms' tumour are children who appear to be healthy and thriving but have an asymptomatic abdominal mass. The tumour is often discovered accidentally by parents or by a physician during a routine physical examination.

Vague abdominal pain, gross haematuria or non-specific symptoms such as malaise, constipation or fever may be seen in 20–30% of children. The acute onset of a complex of symptoms and signs consisting of fever, abdominal mass, anaemia and hypertension points to the diagnosis of Wilms' tumour.

Physical examination generally reveals a smooth, non-tender, firm mass confined to one side of the abdomen. Hypertension may result from encroachment by the tumour on the blood supply to the renal tissue or renin secretion by tumour tissue.

The main difficulty in differential diagnosis lies in distinguishing Wilms' tumour from neuroblastoma.

23.3 HISTOPATHOLOGY

Wilms' tumour is characterized by histological diversity. Most Wilms' tumours are unicentric lesions. The appearance can vary between different parts of the tumour. The classic microscopic pattern is triphasic, which includes blastemal, epithelial and stromal cells. A biphasic pattern or specimens consisting predominantly of one cell type may also be seen in Wilms' tumour. More than 85% of the tumours have favourable histology, and the response of the tumours to treatment is predictable in such cases. The National Wilms' Tumour Study I has identified a sarcomatous or anaplastic variety which responds poorly to treatment and where there is more than 50% mortality. The clear-cell variant of Wilms' tumour has a tendency to metastasize in bones and the rhabdoid variety has a tendency to metastasize in the brain, with development of other central nervous system tumours.

It is also important to distinguish in infancy the tumours called congenital mesoblastic nephroma, in which surgery alone is curative. The association of renal dysplasia with areas of nephroblastomatosis, often bilateral and associated with Beckwith–Weidemann syndrome, requires identification as these are precursors of Wilms' tumour.

23.4 INVESTIGATIONS

Careful physical examination should take note of hemihypertrophy, aniridia or the features of Beckwith–Wiedemann syndrome. All causes of an abdominal mass with or without dilated anterior abdominal veins and abdominal distension must be considered in the differential diagnosis, including neuroblastoma, hydronephrosis, cystic renal disease, splenomegaly, lymphoma and mesenteric cyst. Less common intra-renal neoplasms include mesoblastic nephroma and renal cell carcinoma. Laboratory studies should include a complete blood count, urinalysis and perhaps a spot test for urinary catecholamines. Assessment of liver function and renal function are usually performed pre-operatively for baseline comparison.

Plain abdominal radiograph examination will reveal the presence of a mass with or without calcification. Intravenous urography will show the displacement and distortion of the renal collecting system. It also delineates the opposite kidney. Haemorrhage or necrosis within the tumour may produce radiolucent areas. An inferior venacavogram may provide additional information about tumour extension into the inferior vena cava. Infradiaphragmatic ultra-sonography in conjunction with intravenous urography allows a firm diagnosis to be established and also helps to determine whether there is a tumour thrombus in the ipsilateral or contralateral renal vein or inferior vena cava and whether such thrombi extend into the right atrium. Ultrasonography is of great value in evaluating a child with a non-functioning kidney. An ultrasound scan also detects metastatic involvement in the retroperitoneal lymph node, inferior vena cava and the liver.

Chest roentgenograms will reveal the presence of pulmonary metastasis. Imaging studies of bone and brain are not advocated unless the tumour is found to be a clear-cell sarcoma or rhabdoid tumour.

23.5 STAGING AND PROGNOSIS

The staging of Wilms' tumour is given in Table 23.1.

The extent of disease at diagnosis and at surgery, unfavourable histology and lymph node involvement are the major non-treatment factors that predict prognosis. Certain minor non-treatment factors which affect prognosis are tumour size, age, operative spillage of tumour and invasion of extra-renal vessels within the abdomen.

Table 23.1 Staging of Wilms' tumour

Stage	Definition
I	Tumour is limited to the kidney and completely resected. The surface of the renal capsule is intact. The tumour was not ruptured before or during removal.
II	Tumour extends locally beyond the renal pseudocapsule to involve the renal pelvis, peri-renal soft tissues, peri-aortic lymph nodes and/or the renal vein. There is no residual tumour beyond the margins of resection.
III	Residual non-haematogenous tumour confined to the abdomen resulting from tumour rupture before or during surgery, biopsy of the tumour, tumour implants on the peritoneal surfaces, lymph nodes involved beyond the abdominal peri-aortic chains, and/or tumour incompletely resected because of local infiltration into vital structures.
IV	Haematogenous metastases to lung, liver, bone or brain
V	Bilateral renal involvement either initially or subsequently

Wilms' tumour is the classic example of a tumour where improvement in treatment results has been obtained by optimization of therapy through a multidisciplinary approach and co-operation between paediatric surgeons, radiotherapists, paediatric pathologists and paediatric oncologists.

23.6 TREATMENT – CHOICE OF MODALITY

Surgical extirpation remains the initial treatment for Wilms' tumour. The surgeon's responsibility is to assess the location and extent of the tumour precisely, so it may be accurately staged.

A transverse transperitoneal incision should be made to allow complete exploration of the abdomen. The contralateral kidney should be explored before one proceeds with the dissection of the tumour. *En bloc* excision of the kidney and perinephric extension of tumour, ureter and renal pedicle is done if the tumour is unilateral.

When primary surgery is not possible, pre-operative therapy may be given. Pre-operative chemotherapy reduces the size of large tumours and makes excision less hazardous.

In the case of bilateral tumours, excision (partial nephrectomy) may be undertaken if sufficient renal parenchyma can be preserved on one or either side. If this is not feasible, chemotherapy is administered and second-look surgery is undertaken after 3–4

Table 23.2 Treatment according to stage

Stage	Surgery	Radiotherapy	Chemotherapy
I	Yes	No	Vincristine Actinomycin D
II	Yes	No	Vincristine Actinomycin D
III	Yes	Yes	Vincristine Actinomycin D
IV	Biopsy or resection	Abdominal radiotherapy depending on the extent of the abdominal disease. Radiotherapy of metastatic sites depending on the indication (see text)	As stage III

months. Post-operative treatment depends on the stage and the histology. The general plan according to the stage of the disease is given in Table 23.2.

When radiation is to be given the tumour bed including the whole width of the vertebrae is included in the portal from the 2nd week. The dose is 180 cGy daily to a total dose of 10.8 Gy in 6 fractions to the flank. If there is diffuse peritoneal seeding or massive spillage, whole abdominal X-ray irradiation should be given: 150 cGy daily for 7 fractions to a total dose of 10.5 Gy. If residual disease measuring more than 3 cm is left behind, another boost of 10.8 Gy is given over 6 days to the residual tumour.

The tumour bed is determined by pre-operative intravenous urogram or computed tomographic scan and is defined as the outline of the kidney plus the tumour masses. When whole-abdominal X-ray irradiation is given, the field extends from the diaphragmatic dome to the level of the bottom of the obturator foramina. Femoral heads are shielded from the beam to avoid slipping of the epiphysis.

In stage IV, infradiaphragmatic radiation is given if the primary tumour would otherwise have qualified as in stage III. Non-resectable metastases in liver are treated with radiotherapy with 2 cm margins. If there are pulmonary metastases both lungs are treated with X-ray irradiation from apex to base with humoral head shielding. The dose is 12 Gy in 8 fractions and a boost of 7.5 Gy in 5 fractions is given to the site of metastasis. Chemotherapy with three drugs is given for 65 weeks as per the stage III schedule.

Table 23.3 Age-adjusted dosage for stage II–IV tumours

Age of patient (months)	Total dose (Gy)
0–12	14.4
13–18	21.6
19–30	27
31–40	32.4
≥ 41	37.8

23.6.1 Anaplastic Wilms' tumour

Stage I tumours are treated just like stage I tumours with favourable histology and no routine radiation is given. Stage II, III and IV receive X-ray irradiation for those with favourable histology but they should receive age-adjusted doses as shown in Table 23.3.

23.6.2 Clear-cell sarcoma of the kidney

All patients should receive post-operative radiotherapy to the tumour bed as described for tumours with favourable histology.

23.6.3 Bilateral

Prognosis depends on the extent of disease. Excision is performed at the initial operation only if all the tumour can be removed with preservation of sufficient renal parenchyma on one or both sides. Chemotherapy of VCDA is given as previously described. After three months patients are re-evaluated and if the lesion is found to be resectable, it should be resected. If there is no residual disease, chemotherapy is to be continued. If there is demonstrable disease, radiotherapy should be added.

24

Neuroblastoma

Neuroblastoma is one of the tumours that originate in the neural crest cells that give rise to the sympathetic nervous system. It is one of the most biologically remarkable tumours of childhood. Neuroblastoma has the highest rate of spontaneous remission described for any malignant neoplasm. It also demonstrates spontaneous and induced maturation. In no other tumour is age of such profound importance in prognosis. Maximum survival is seen among children less than one year old regardless of the extent of the tumour at the time of diagnosis.

24.1 INCIDENCE AND RISK FACTORS

Neuroblastoma is the most common extracranial malignant solid tumour of childhood (7.8%) and occurs slighty more frequently in boys. The median age at diagnosis is less than two years old with 35% of the children less than one year old, 55% less than two years old and 88% less than five years old. The tumour may occur in the intra-uterine fetus, occasionally with metastasis to the placenta. The aetiology of neuroblastoma is unknown. Neuroblastoma has been observed with increased frequency in patients with neurofibromatosis, Beckwith–Wiedemann syndrome and nisidiroblastosis. It has been associated in several cases with the fetal hydantoin syndrome.

Cytogenetic studies of neuroblastoma cells have demonstrated abnormalities in approximately 80% of cases. The oncogenes N-*myx* and N-*ras* are amplified in neuroblastoma cells. N-*myc* DNA amplification and RNA expression have been reported to increase with tumour progression.

24.2 PRESENTATION AND NATURAL HISTORY

Neuroblastoma may originate anywhere along the sympathetic nervous system. The most common site of primary tumour is within the abdomen (70%) – either in the adrenal gland (40%) or in a paraganglion, visceral ganglia and abdominal side chain. The remaining 30% originate in the cervical, thoracic and pelvic side chains. A small proportion of patients do not have any discernible primary tumour at diagnosis. Approximately 50% of infants (< 5 years old) and 70% of older children present with evidence of tumour spread beyond the primary site. Multiple primary tumours can also occur.

Presenting signs and symptoms differ depending on the primary site and site of metastasis. A cervical mass may be associated with Horner's syndrome and heterochromia of the iris, respiratory distress and infection, dysphagia and circulatory problems. A lower thoracic tumour may not produce many symptoms. An abdominal mass that produces stretching or compression of the renal vasculature can result in severe hypertension. Paraspinal tumours at any site may extend through the spinal foramina with subsequent cord compression (dumbell tumour). In infants, diffuse liver metastasis can lead to an enlarged liver and give rise to prolonged jaundice and circulatory problems. Subcutaneous metastases appear as nontender, bluish, mobile nodules. The older age group shows a different pattern of metastatic spread. Skeletal bone marrow and lymph node metastases are predominant in this age group. The tendency to skeletal spread is particularly evident in the skull and facial bones, especially in the orbits, which can give rise to proptosis and to ecchymosis in the upper eye lid. The bone pain and signs may resemble those of rheumatic fever or leukaemia. Lymph node metastases are also frequent.

24.3 HISTOPATHOLOGY

Neuroblastoma is derived from the primitive stem cells that differentiate into sympathoblasts. The primitive stem cells may also differentiate into paragangliomas. Neuroblastoma is a round-cell tumour of childhood. An undifferentiated neuroblastoma consists of closely packed small round cells without any special arrangement or differentiation. The nuclei are hyperchromatic. As maturation occurs, cells begin to differentiate to ganglioma cells. Uniform maturation occurs or there may be areas of maturation interspersed with areas of undifferentiated cells (ganglioneuroblastoma). Completely differentiated cells form the ganglioneuroma with well-differentiated ganglion cells, Schwann cells and nerve bundles.

24.4 INVESTIGATIONS

The work-up should include a complete blood count, liver and kidney function studies, and urine assay for catecholamine metabolites. Diagnostic imaging studies include chest radiograph, abdominal radiograph, skeletal survey, bone marrow aspiration and biopsy.

24.5 STAGING AND PROGNOSIS

The classic staging system used in neuroblastoma is that proposed by Evans *et al.* in 1971 (Table 24.1). Tumour resectability is not incorporated in this staging system. Other staging systems exist.

The prognosis is best when the patient presents in the early stages.

Table 24.1 Clinical staging system proposed by Evans *et al.*

Stage	Definition
I	Tumour is confined to the organ or structure of origin
II	Tumour extends in continuity beyond the organ or structure of origin but does not cross the midline. Regional lymph nodes on the same side may be involved. For tumours arising on the midline structures, penetration beyond the capsule and/or involvement of lymph nodes shall be considered stage II.
III	Tumour extends in continuity beyond the midline; regional nodes may be involved bilaterally
IV	Remote disease involves skeleton, organs, soft tissue, distant nodes
IV–S	Patients would otherwise be stage I or II but have remote disease confined only to one or more of the following sites: liver, skin or bone marrow (but not bone).

24.6 TREATMENT – CHOICE OF MODALITY

24.6.1 Surgery

Surgery alone may be curative in this condition. The role of surgery is both diagnostic and therapeutic. Complete removal of the tumour offers the best chance for cure. This is possible mostly in stages I and II. It must be established pre-operatively wehther the disease is clinically localized or distant disease is present. Initially, control by chemotherapy or radiotherapy is impossible and an attempt at resection should be made approximately four months later. At the time of second-look procedure, complete excision is possible in about 50% of these patients.

Patients with localized disease arising in the thorax appear to have good prognosis and surgical removal is always worthwhile in these cases. Lymph node sampling is carried out in all cases unless precluded by the size and extent of the tumour.

24.6.2 Radiotherapy

Radiotherapy is a major component of multidisciplinary treatment for neuroblastoma. The therapeutic dose usually delivered ranges from 15 to 35 Gy depending on the age of the child and the site being irradiated. It is the primary method of treatment for unresectable tumour in the neck and upper thorax.

In extensive regional disease, pre-operative or post-operative radiotherapy may increase the chance for cure. In more critical situations such as spinal cord compression by tumour or loss of vision with orbital metastasis, radiotherapy is a very effective form of treatment which may restore the functions rapidly. Radiotherapy is also effective for pain control in patients who have symptomatic bone lesions.

24.6.3 Chemotherapy

Vincristine, adriamycin, endoxan and DTIC are useful in neuroblastoma, and *cis*-platin and holoxan are also being evaluated. In early-stage disease where surgical excision had been complete, adjuvant chemotherapy has not improved the treatment results.

Chemotherapy in advanced cases has not produced any impressive cure rates. It has helped to reduce bulky disease in inoperable cases to operable stage. In stage III disease, chemotherapy has marginally improved cure rates when used pre-operatively and post-operatively with radiation.

25

Skin

25.1 INCIDENCE AND RISK FACTORS

The incidence of malignant cutaneous epitheliomas relates to environmental conditions and to the occupation and pigmentation of the patient.

In many tropical and subtropical areas, the highest prevalence of non-melanomatous skin cancer is among fair-skinned people. Lesions predominantly occur in areas of chronic solar dermatitis. Solar-related skin cancers are generally the most common neoplasms among white populations living close to the equator. Among populations with various degrees of skin pigmentation (melanin), those with the deepest pigmentation have the lowest incidence of skin cancer. This confirms the supposition that melanin protects the skin from harmful ultraviolet waves.

However, in rural populations there is an incidence of cancer in the lower extremities that appears to be related to chronic skin ulcers from a variety of causes, including burns. These lesions are exclusively squamous cell carcinoma (in contrast to the predominant basal cell carcinoma seen in white populations). These lesions are often advanced, with deep invasion of adjacent tissues and regional lymph node metastases. In contrast, basal cell carcinomas rarely metastasize.

Skin cancers can be generally subdivided into melanomatous and non-melanomatous malignant lesions. The best method of management of melanomas is universally accepted to be surgical and will not be discussed.

25.2 PRESENTATION AND NATURAL HISTORY

An understanding of the origin of malignant neoplasms of the skin and of approaches to treatment is aided by knowledge of the skin's basic structure. The epidermis varies in thickness from 60 μm (0.06 mm) in the eyelid and vulva to 1 mm in exposed sites such as the palms and soles. Epidermal cells extend into the dermis (dense connective tissue) and occasionally into the looser subcutaneous connective tissue, and include those of the fat and sweat glands and the hair follicles. They have an important role in re-epithelialization of the epidermis after injury. Epithelial outgrowth is often noted from sites of hair follicles and sweat glands after superficial desquamation following thermal burns or radiation therapy. The incidence of basal cell carcinomas has been correlated with the incidence of sebaceous glands.

25.3 HISTOPATHOLOGY

Skin epitheliomas are divided into basal cell and squamous cell carcinomas.

25.4 INVESTIGATIONS

Standard inspection of the skin in populations at risk is one of the simplest parts of the physical examination.

Epitheliomas are characterized by raised, sometimes ulcerated lesions, often with pearly margins and rather firm consistency. Any non-healing ulcerated lesion is suspicious and should be examined and if necessary biopsied at an early stage.

Distinction from typical tropical lesions such as yaws and other tropical ulcers due to infections is based on lack of response to appropriate antibiotic therapy.

25.5 STAGING AND PROGNOSIS

Assessment of the stage of skin cancer is based on inspection and palpation of the involved area and the regional lymph nodes. Occasionally, radiographic studies of bony structures underlying

Table 25.1 Classifications of skin cancer

Stage	Definition
Primary tumour (T)	
TI	Tumour $\leqslant$ 2 cm in greatest dimension
T2	Tumour 2–5 cm in greatest dimension
T3	Tumour $>$ 5 cm in greatest dimension
T4	Tumour invades deep extradermal structures, e.g. cartilage, skeletal muscle, bone
Lymph node (N)	
Nx	Regional lymph nodes cannot be assessed
N0	No regional lymph node metastases
N1	Regional lymph node metastases
Distant metastasis (M)	
Mx	Presence of distant metastases cannot be assessed
M0	No distant metastases
M1	Distant metastases

Table 25.2 Stage grouping

Stage	TNM classification		
I	T1	N0	M0
II	T2–T3	N0	M0
III	T4	N0	M0
	Any T	N1	M0
IV	Any T	Any N	M1

advanced lesions are necessary. The classifications used are shown in Tables 25.1 and 25.2.

25.6 TREATMENT – CHOICE OF MODALITY

Normally T1 and T2 epitheliomas are readily curable by excision, radiotherapy or other procedures such as cryosurgery, laser therapy, and diathermy and curettage. The earliest epitheliomas which may in fact be keratoses can be treated by simple electrodessication with or without curettage. These are important measures in populations with multiple lesions, but such management is labour-intensive. The use of 5-fluorouracil 5% ointment is useful for patients with widespread premalignant changes. The application of this ointment twice daily for six weeks will eliminate most keratoses and superficial epitheliomas and leave deeper epitheliomas more obvious with erythema and occasional oedema which will pinpoint them for further definitive therapy by excision or radiotherapy.

25.6.1 Radical (curative) radiotherapy

(a) Physical considerations (photon beams)

Cutaneous cancer grows on the body surface and only rarely is it accessible from an opposing surface (such as in an earlobe). The majority of techniques therefore depend on a single incident beam of radiation. Massive involvement may justify angled beams with wedges. The goal is to limit the radiation entirely to the tumour-bearing area. A practical compromise is to select those physical factors, including radiation quality, source–tumour distance and radiation area, which will encompass the lateral limits of the tumour with its estimated microscopic extension and limit transmitted radiation to underlying structures to a minimum. To accomplish this requires an accurate assessment of gross tumour extent by means of measurement with ruler or callipers, estimation of microscopic invasion and depth by examination of an adequate biopsy of the margins, and other clinical aids such as roentgenograms. Electron beams will achieve this aim with greatest success when lesions are limited to within a few centimetres of the surface. At present, however, only radiograph and gamma beams of selected energy and focal distance are available in the majority of radiotherapy departments.

Beginning with an energy level of about 30 kV a fairly continuous spectrum of radiograph beams of energy ranging up to the megavoltage region should provide an adequate armamentarium for all possible situations. Lesions ranging in depth from a few millimetres to several centimetres can thus be effectively radiated with fair homogeneity of dose within the tumour and with reasonable limitation of transmitted dose.

The ideal conditions of limiting the radiation to the tumour volume alone cannot be achieved by external X-ray irradiation. The judicious selection of treatment factors and shielding will minimize transmitted irradiation. However, the eye, middle ear and brain must be considered special problems and elaborate measures should be undertaken to reduce the dose to the absolute minimum in these sites. The generally accepted maximally tolerated dose to the lens is 5 Gy, and that to the brain is 50 Gy over a protracted course of treatment of 5–6 weeks. A relative contra-indication to radiation therapy exists if adequate protection to these or other vital structures is not possible.

Other irradiation modalities include interstitial gamma irradiation, external short-distance gamma irradiation, and electron-beam irradiation. Only the last agent is likely to demonstrate physical advantages over external X-ray irradiation of using a suitable combination of factors.

(b) Collimation of external beams

The irradiation margins should be determined by clinical judgement. A fixed margin around visible or palpable tumours such as 0.5 or 1 cm may needlessly irradiate normal tissue in some instances of small and non-infiltrating tumours while undertreating others that may be large and widely infiltrating as determined by clinical and histological examination.

It makes good sense, radiobiologically, to deliver two-thirds to three-quarters of the dosage to the tumour and its margin, then to reduce the treatment area to circumscribe only the clinical tumour for the full dosage. This is based on the anticipated higher sensitivity of microscopic nests of tumour cells because of lower cell number and better oxygenation. This 'controlled penumbra' form of treatment reduces the normal tissue dosage and should therefore give improved cosmetic results. It is of vital importance to shield underlying structures whenever possible, as shown in Figure 25.1. This should be done even when optimum depth–dose distribution can be obtained, because any transmitted irradiation is unnecessary radiation. In sites where underlying structures cannot be shielded, special precautions should be made to select the best possible quality of irradiation that will minimize the transmitted dose.

The treatment volume should be shaped to the tumour and its margin. This is most easily accomplished by tracing the field on transparent film or cellophane and transferring the pattern to a lead shield of a thickness not transmitting more than 5% irradiation. A treatment cone alone should not be used because patient movement may result in geometric miss. It is far better to construct a special shield or a lead face mask which is fixed to the patient, and to treat through the resulting aperture with a generously wide beam.

(c) Dosage

The dose necessary to cure skin cancer increases with the volume (or area) of the cancer. Thus a small flat lesion of less than 1 cm diameter can be cured by a single dose of 27–30 Gy. However, the

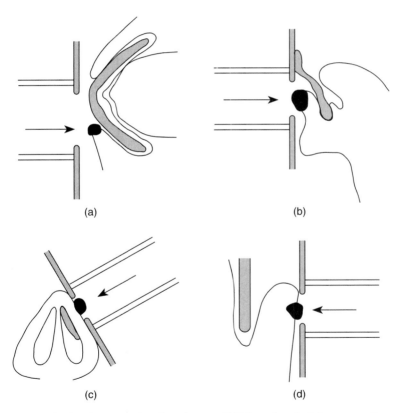

(a)

(b)

(c)

(d)

Figure 25.1 Diagrams showing the possibilities of underlying as well as peripheral protection in radiation therapy of tumours of (a) the eyelid , (b) the lip, (c) the nose, and (d) the ear. The lead shielding should be coated with paraffin or plastic. Lead rubber is also useful. The shielding is shown as shaded areas.

Table 25.3 Recommended dosage

Diameter of field (cm)	Minimum number of fractions	Total dose (Gy)	Dose per fraction (Gy)
< 1	1	27–30	27–30
1–2	5	36–40	7.2–8
2–3	10	40–43	4–4.5
3–4	15	43–47	2.9–3.1
> 4	20	46–51	2.3–2.5

cosmetic result is better if the dose is fractionated. If this is logistically feasible, the treatments should be fractionated over a week or two. The number of fractions must increase with larger fields in order to present good cosmetic function. Table 25.3 shows the recommended number of fractions and total dosage, based on experience.

(d) Benign lesions

Two significant benign lesions are also often treated by radiation therapy: keloids and keratoacanthoma.

Keloids

These lesions are particularly common in Africa and they often become large and symptomatic. Such lesions have been treated by surgical excision but the recurrence rate is high. It has been found that post-operative radiation therapy is effective in eliminating or reducing the recurrence of these lesions.

Radiation therapy alone is effective only in the treatment of quite small and fresh keloids. Therefore, the general treatment of choice is surgical excision followed by immediate radiation therapy. It is probable that the time-lag between surgery and radiation should not be longer than 48 hours and that treatment on the same day is both logistically sensible and most effective. A single dose is nearly always satisfactory. The preferred dose recommended by many is 12 Gy, with some increase for unusually large keloids. The technique is to give a reasonable margin of 1 cm around the excision site and to treat with superficial radiation, ranging from 50–200 kV depending on the thickness of the skin.

Keratoacanthoma

The cause of this lesion is still unknown, although association with chemicals such as oils in industry, trauma or actinic exposure has been found. Clinical diagnosis is possible because of the unusual natural history of keratoacanthoma. The lesion often starts as a papule and reaches 1–2 cm in diameter within weeks. The tumour has a central umbilication and ulceration. Lesions that have been treated conservatively with observation only have often grown large and led to destruction of nearby tissues, requiring later major resection and reconstructive surgery. This fact outweighs the occasional spontaneous regression of keratoacanthoma and indicates the need for early treatment. They have been found to be quite radiosensitive, probably more so than malignant epitheliomas. Therefore, early treatment with radiation therapy is indicated. In general, a dose of about three-quarters of the dose normally used for treatment of a malignant epithelioma can be used.

Kaposi's sarcoma

This lesion is a major component of the AIDS complex. Malignant disseminated Kaposi's sarcoma is dealt with in Chapter 26.

25.6.2 Palliative radiotherapy

There is a point beyond which skin cancer cannot be cured, for example when there is massive local invasion of underlying structures including bone and the presence of large and/or multiple regional lymph node metastases. Radiation can provide palliation for painful ulcers, bleeding and sepsis on occasions, but supportive care including antibiotics and analgesics is more important. The shortest possible treatment usually at a dose of approximately two-thirds of the curative dose and over fewer fractions may be provided in addition to the all-important supportive care.

26

AIDS-related cancers

26.1 INCIDENCE AND RISK FACTORS

AIDS is a major worldwide epidemic. From the small numbers of cases recognized in 1982, the figures rose to 2.5 million persons infected with HIV in the USA alone in 1990. The highest rates are in sub-Saharan Africa where many millions are infected, Zambia, Tanzania, Uganda, Rwanda, Burundi and Zimbabwe having probably the highest incidence rates. In all these countries the incidence of HIV infection amongst prostitutes and in the armed forces is even higher.

About 40% of patients with AIDS will develop a malignancy, usually Kaposi's sarcoma (KS) or a B-cell lymphoma. Therefore, a huge increase in the numbers of KS and non-Hodgkin's lymphomas is expected in all these countries. Evidence of such an increase has been seen.

KAPOSI'S SARCOMA

26.2 PRESENTATION AND NATURAL HISTORY

There are five manifestations of KS, as shown in Table 26.1. The classic kind was first described in Eastern European Jewish men and is indolent, rarely causing death. The African kind is more aggressive. A visceral variant (not uncommon in children), affecting viscera and often lymph nodes, runs a shorter course. A fourth kind occurs in renal transplant patients and principally affects the lower limbs, is equally common in men and women, and sometimes regresses after cessation of immunosuppressive treatment. The fifth

Table 26.1 Comparison of the clinical features of the different forms of Kaposi's sarcoma

Type	Patient characteristics	Clinical presentation	Prognosis
Classic	Age 50–70 years; male:female ratio 10:1; Jewish or Italian	Lower limbs, slow progression, gradual local spread, oedema	Good, 8–12 years; death from other causes
African (locally aggressive)	Age 20–50 years; blacks; central and southern Africa	Localized florid nodules or infiltrative lesions	Survive for 5–8 years
African (visceral)	Black; children; male:female ratio 3:1	Viscera and lymph nodes involved	Usually die within 3 years
Renal transplant	Mean 17 months after transplant; male:female ratio 3:1	Cutaneous, usually legs; 30% have more aggressive form	Variable, may respond to change in immunosuppression
Epidemic	Homosexuals, drug addicts, haemophiliacs, sexual partners of HIV-positive people	Widespread cutaneous and/or visceral disease	Very poor, deaths often from opportunistic infections

kind, epidemic KS (EKS), may vary in intensity from a benign disease which does not progress over many months to a fulminating systemic disease which is rapidly fatal. EKS affects between a third and a quarter of all homosexual AIDS patients in Western countries, while the disease is seen in heterosexuals with AIDS in Africa.

The commonest presentation of EKS is of several lesions occurring within a short time, sometimes in crops. This is usually seen in the trunk or limbs, but the head and neck may be affected, especially the palate or nose. Nodules may also develop at sites of previous trauma (Koebner's phenomenon) or along skin creases (Langer's lines). The legs can become oedematous or thickened, with ulceration, pain and secondary infection. Five per cent of patients have visceral or nodal disease without cutaneous involvement, while 30% have localized lesions only. However, assessments of the frequency of visceral disease depend on the rigour with which it is sought. The gastrointestinal tract is second only to the skin in frequency of KS. Part of the bowel is affected in 45% of EKS patients.

KS in the oral cavity is easily detected. The lesions start as reddish or purple macules, coalescing into nodules or plaques. Pulmonary KS occurs in about 10% of cases and has a very poor

Table 26.2 Krigel's staging system

Stage	Definition
I	Locally indolent cutaneous disease
II	Cutaneous disease that is locally aggressive or where there is associated lymphadenopathy
III	Generalized disease involving skin or mucous membranes and/or involvement of axillary or inguinal lymph nodes
IV	Visceral involvement with greater than 5 GI lesions or combined diameter of visceral lesions greater than 5 cm

prognosis. A chest radiograph may show diffuse pulmonary infiltration, pleural effusion or hilar lymphadenopathy. Obstruction of the respiratory tract can occur at any level from the larynx down to the smaller bronchi. Lymph node involvement occurs in 40–50% of EKS cases and can lead to a diagnostic problem since progressive generalized lymphadenopathy or infections causing lymph node enlargement commonly occur in patients with EKS.

EKS is not commonly the cause of death in AIDS patients – only 15% of KS patients die of their sarcoma while 85% die of opportunistic infections, and other causes.

26.3 HISTOPATHOLOGY

The pathology of KS is the same for all clinical and epidemiological varieties of the disease. Initial abnormal dilated blood vessels in the dermis lead to the formation of irregular vascular slits with an inflammatory infiltrate of lymphocytes, plasma cells and other mononuclear cells.

26.4 INVESTIGATIONS

Full blood count. liver function tests and chest radiograph should be performed, as well as a radiograph of the affected limbs if there is any suggestion of bony involvement.

26.5 STAGING AND PROGNOSIS

The staging system for EKS is shown in Table 26.2.

There is a clear correlation between stage and prognosis. The extent of Kaposi's sarcoma reflects the immune status of the patient and early stages have a better prognosis. Patients with visceral disease show only 25% of the survival of those without, and pulmonary involvement is especially ominous.

26.6 TREATMENT – CHOICE OF MODALITY

26.6.1 Radiotherapy

EKS is not generally life-threatening, but can be in the case of respiratory or massive intra-abdominal disease. Treatment should therefore be tailored to suit the form of the disease. Lesions of EKS are not as radiosensitive as the classic variety, although the evidence is conflicting. A single fraction of 8 Gy with 100 KV will produce partial response but will only rarely eradicate the lesion. The relapse rate is high in patients surviving long enough, so that many patients require a second treatment. Bleeding lesions of the feet, penis or palate resolve readily using 20 Gy/5 fr/1 week, preventing an infective hazard to contacts and staff. Ulcerated palatal lesions also resolve readily, as does periorbital oedema with local radiotherapy.

With more widespread lesions, hemi-body radiation may be used, e.g. 7–8 Gy to the lower half or 6 Gy to the upper half with megavoltage using full bolus. Patients need anti-emetics and often require overnight admission with the upper hemi-body treatment. Where there is considerable oedema, a fractionated course, e.g. 20 Gy/5 fr or even 30 Gy/10 fr, is better. Electrons are appropriate and total-body electron therapy to a dose of 25 Gy/10 fr/5 weeks may be used if available.

26.6.2 Chemotherapy

Chemotherapy is very effective in classic KS, notably vinblastine, actinomycin D, vincristine, bleomycin, and dacarbazine, with complete response rates of 20–40% and overall response rates of 58–88% reported.

However, the role of chemotherapy in EKS is less clear. These patients are immunosuppressed, often neutropenic or thrombocytopenic, and develop more marked side-effects to chemotherapy than non-AIDS patients. Steroids, because of their immuno-suppressive effects, should not be used in patients with AIDS. Etoposide and vinblastine give 70% and 25–60% response rates, respectively, but are myelosuppressive. Vincristine gives a 45% response rate and is less marrow-toxic, but patients with HIV infection have an increased susceptibility to the development of neurotoxicity. A recently developed regime is vincristine 2 mg and bleomycin 30 mg both given intravenously as a 24 h infusion every three weeks.

Intralesional chemotherapy with vinblastine has been used but is painful and gives similar results to 100 kV X-rays. Interferon therapy causes less severe immunodeficiency and results in less severe opportunistic infections than chemotherapy. However, high-dose interferon is necessary, with considerable side-effects: shivering, fevers and malaise.

The basic problem with both chemotherapy and immunotherapy in EKS is expense. For developing countries, both these methods of treatment should be avoided and the mainstay of treatment should be radiotherapy and palliative care.

26.7 OUTCOME

Since AIDS is a fatal illness, all treatment is palliative. However, radiotherapy produces excellent responses, either complete or par-tial. Difficulties may arise in the definition of response, since lesions may regress but leave residual pigmentation. Side-effects to radio-therapy are more marked in AIDS patients than in non-AIDS patients, thus influencing treatment planning.

NON-HODGKIN'S LYMPHOMA

26.8 PRESENTATION AND NATURAL HISTORY

This HIV-related B-cell lymphoma in Western countries is seen in homosexual men rather than in other risk groups such as haemo-philiacs and intravenous drug abusers. The lymphoma is often advanced at presentation and B symptoms of fever and weight loss are frequent. About 50% of patients give a history of previous opportunistic infection.

26.9 HISTOPATHOLOGY

Several characteristics distinguish HIV-related lymphoma from non-HIV-related lymphoma:

- commonly extranodal: 67% are purely extranodal, while 9% have some involvement of extranodal sites, especially central nervous system, bone marrow, gastrointestinal tract including rectum. and mucocutaneous sites;
- high incidence of primary brain lymphomas: these represent 20% of AIDS lymphomas; and
- commonly high-grade (over 60%), especially of small non-cleaved (Burkitt's or non-Burkitt's) or immunoblastic type.

The lymphoma must be distinguished from the progressive generalized lymphadenopathy commonly seen in AIDS patients, and central nervous system lymphomas must be differentiated from infections of the nervous system common in AIDS, and also from AIDS-related dementia. In progressive generalized lymphadenopathy, there is extensive follicular hyperplasia and plasmacytosis of lymph nodes, with a polyclonal rise in serum immunoglobulins. A rapid rise in nodal size or the development of B symptoms may herald the progression to lymphoma.

26.10 INVESTIGATIONS

A limited staging procedure should be done: radiograph of chest and affected sites, bone marrow aspirate and trephine, liver scan or ultrasound. A computed tomographic scan of the abdomen and pelvis should be obtained when available. Immunoglobulin and liver function tests should be performed, and full blood count erythrocytic sedimentation rate, and the size of all node masses recorded.

26.11 STAGING AND PROGNOSIS

Stage for stage, HIV-related lymphomas have a worse prognosis than non-HIV-related lymphomas. This is especially so in the central nervous system. The responses to treatment are very short-lived in patients with HIV-related lymphoma. The survival for these patients is dismal: about three months for high-grade lymphoma, and six months for intermediate-grade lymphoma.

26.12 TREATMENT – CHOICE OF MODALITY

HIV-related lymphoma is often a fatal illness which requires active treatment. A minority have low-grade lymphomas which should be treated by radiotherapy. Patients with primary brain lymphomas should also be treated with radiotherapy, keeping chemotherapy in reserve for relapse. The standard dose for radiotherapy is 30–40 Gy/ 15–20 fr/3–4 weeks.

High-grade lymphomas are more difficult to treat. Aggressive combination chemotherapy has led to complete responses rates of 50–60% in Western countries, but relapse occurs early, especially in the central nervous system, and prolongation of survival is rare. Since these patients do not have a long life-span ahead, it is best to use less aggressive regimes for palliation.

26.13 OUTCOME

Results in cerebral HIV-related lymphoma are very discouraging. Many brain lymphomas progress during radiotherapy, and do not show the radiosensitivity of non-HIV-related brain lymphoma. AIDS patients with lymphoma outside the central nervous system fare better than those with lymphoma within the central nervous system, although less well than non-AIDS patients with lymphomas.

26.14 MORBIDITY

HIV patients have an increased morbidity to radiotherapy or chemo-therapy, for the same treatment, compared with non-HIV patients.

26.15 PALLIATIVE TREATMENT

Short courses of palliative radiotherapy are of value in HIV-related lymphoma for diminishing tumour size, and relieving obstruction, headache, etc. due to incurable tumour. Doses of 10 Gy/1 fr to 25 Gy/5 fr can be used.

Counselling is of great importance in caring for AIDS patients. The patients must not be allowed to feel isolated. As far as possible, the patient should be allowed to stay at home for the terminal phase. It should be explained to the family that the infectivity of HIV through casual contact is very low. Cutlery and towels, etc. can be shared, except when the patient has an obviously discharging lesion.

References

Dukes, C.E. (1932) The classification of cancer of the rectum. *Journal of Pathology and Bacteriology*, **35**, 322–32.

Hall, E.J. (1994) *Radiobiology for the Radiologist*, 4th edn, J.B. Lippincott, Philadelphia.

ICRU (1993) Prescribing, recording and reporting photon beam therapy. *ICRU Report No. 50*, International Commission on Radiation Units and Measurements, Bethesda, Maryland, USA.

Russell, W.O., Chen, J., Enzinger, F. *et al.* (1977) A clinical and pathological staging system for soft tissue sarcomas. *Cancer*, **40**, 1562–70.

World Health Organization (1995) *National Cancer Control Programmes: Priorities and Managerial Guidelines*, World Health Organization, Geneva.

Zulch, K.J. (1979) Histological typing of tumours of the central nervous system. *International Histological Classification of Tumours, No. 21*, World Health Organization, Geneva.

Recommended reading

Miller, A.B. (1991) *Cancer Screening*, Cambridge University Press, Cambridge.

Schottenfeld, D. and Fraumeni, J. (1982) *Cancer Epidemiology and Prevention*, W.B. Saunders, Philadelphia.

International Union against Cancer (1993) *Manual of Clinical Oncology*, 7th edn.

World Health Organization (1980) *Optimization of Radiotherapy. WHO Tech. Rep. Ser. 644.*

World Health Organization (1983) *Smoking Control Strategies in Developing Countries. WHO Tech. Rep. Ser. 695.*

World Health Organization (1985) Essential drugs for cancer chemotherapy. Bulletin of the WHO, **63**(6), 999–1002.

World Health Organization (1986) *Cancer Pain Relief*, World Health Organization, Geneva.

World Health Organization (1990) *Cancer Pain Relief and Palliative Care. WHO Tech. Rep. Ser. 804.*

World Health Organization (1992) *Cervical Cancer Screenings Programmes: Management Guidelines*, World Health Organization, Geneva.

Index

Page numbers appearing in *italics* refer to tables; page numbers appearing in **bold** refer to figures